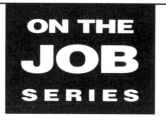

REAL PEOPLE WORKING in

THE HELPING PROFESSIONS

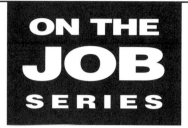

ON THE JOB SERIES

REAL PEOPLE WORKING *in*

THE HELPING PROFESSIONS

Blythe Camenson

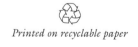

Printed on recyclable paper

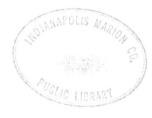

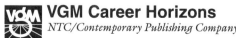

VGM Career Horizons
NTC/Contemporary Publishing Company

Library of Congress Cataloging-in-Publication Data

Camenson, Blythe.
   Real people working in the helping professions / Blythe Camenson.
      p.   cm.—(On the job series)
    ISBN 0-8442-4721-9 (cloth).—ISBN 0-8442-4722-7 (pbk.)
     1. Human services—Vocational guidance—United States. 2. Mental
health services—Vocational guidance—United States. I. Title.
   II. Series: On the job (Lincolnwood, Ill.)
   HV10.5.C35 1997
   361′.0023′73—dc21   97-23005
                                             CIP

Published by VGM Career Horizons
An imprint of NTC/Contemporary Publishing Company
4255 West Touhy Avenue, Lincolnwood (Chicago), Illinois 60646-1975 U.S.A.
Copyright © 1998 by NTC/Contemporary Publishing Company
Printed in the United States of America
International Standard Book Number: 0-8442-4721-9 (cloth)
                                       0-8442-4722-7 (paper)
15   14   13   12   11   10   9   8   7   6   5   4   3   2   1

To Ellen Raphaeli,
advisor, big sister, treasured friend

SO

Contents

Acknowledgments xi

How to Use This Book xiii

Introduction to the Field xv

1. Human Services Workers 1

Overview 1

Training 2

Job Outlook 4

Salaries 5

Related Fields 5

Interview: M. Allen Broyles—Residential
Counselor 6

For More Information 9

2. Social Workers 11

Overview 11

Training 14

Job Outlook 15

Salaries 17

Related Fields 17

Interview: Patricia Morin—Clinical Social Worker 17

For More Information 21

3. Mental Health and Rehabilitation Counselors 23

Overview 23

Training 24

Job Outlook   27

Salaries   27

Related Fields   28

Interview: Romney Latko—Marriage, Family, and
   Child Counselor Trainee   28

Interview: Jane E. Bennett—Vocational
   Rehabilitation Counselor   31

For More Information   34

4. School, College, and Career Counselors   37

Overview   37

Training   38

Job Outlook   39

Salaries   40

Related Fields   40

Interview: Terrence Place—High School Guidance
   Counselor   40

Interview: Cheryl Trull—Adult Education Counselor   43

For More Information   46

5. Special Education   47

Overview   47

Training   49

Job Outlook   51

Salaries   52

Related Fields   52

Interview: Maureen Wright—Teacher of the
   Visually Handicapped   53

Interview: Janice M. Lee—Specialist for the
   Learning Disabled (Graduate Intern)   55

Interview: Lynne Robbins—Elementary Special
   Education Teacher   60

Interview: Elyse Feldman—Educational Therapist   64

For More Information   68

6. Psychologists   69

Overview   69

Training   72

Job Outlook   75

Salaries   77

Related Fields   78

Interview: Gerald D. Oster—Clinical Psychologist   78

Interview: Denise Stybr—School Psychologist   83

For More Information   85

7. Psychiatrists   87

Overview   87

Training   88

Job Outlook   88

Salaries   89

Related Fields   90

Interview: Gerald Horne—Psychiatrist   90

For More Information   92

8. Psychiatric Nurses   95

Overview   95

Training   96

Job Outlook   98

Salaries   99

Related Fields   99

Interview: Monica James—Counselor/Nurse   100

Interview: Rob Verner—Psychiatric Nurse   102

For More Information   104

9. Physical and Occupational Therapists   107

Overview   107

Settings for Physical Therapists   108

Training for Physical Therapists 109

Salaries for the Physical Therapy Profession 110

Job Outlook for Physical Therapists 111

Settings for Occupational Therapists 111

Training for Occupational Therapists 112

Salaries for the Occupational Therapy Profession 113

Related Fields 113

Interview: Laurie DeJong—Physical Therapist 113

Interview: Helen Cox—Occupational Therapist 115

For More Information 117

10. Speech-Language Pathologists and Audiologists 119

Overview 119

Job Settings 123

Training and Qualifications 125

Job Outlook 127

Salaries 128

Related Fields 129

Interview: Fay Dudley—Speech-Language Pathologist 129

For More Information 132

11. Funeral Directors 133

Overview 133

Training 135

Job Outlook 137

Salaries 138

Related Fields 138

Interview: R. Todd Noecker—Funeral Director and Embalmer 138

For More Information 141

About the Author 143

Acknowledgments

The author would like to thank the following professionals for providing information about their careers:

- Jane E. Bennett, vocational rehabilitation counselor

- M. Allen Broyles, residential counselor

- Helen Cox, occupational therapist

- Laurie DeJong, physical therapist

- Fay Dudley, speech-language pathologist

- Elyse Feldman, educational therapist

- Gerald Horne, psychiatrist

- Monica James, counselor/nurse

- Romney Latko, marriage, family, and child counselor trainee

- Janice M. Lee, specialist for the learning disabled (graduate intern)

- Patricia Morin, clinical social worker

- R. Todd Noecker, funeral director

- Gerald D. Oster, clinical psychologist

- Terrence Place, high school guidance counselor

- Lynne Robbins, elementary special education teacher

- Denise Stybr, school psychologist

- Cheryl Trull, adult education counselor

- Rob Verner, psychiatric nurse

- Maureen Wright, teacher of the visually handicapped

How to Use This Book

On the Job: Real People Working in the Helping Professions is part of a series of career books designed to help you find essential information quickly and easily. Unlike other career resources on the market, books in the *On the Job* series provide you with information on hundreds of careers, in an easy-to-use format. This includes information on:

- The nature of the work
- Working conditions
- Employment
- Training, other qualifications, and advancement
- Job outlooks
- Earnings
- Related occupations
- Sources of additional information

But that's not all. You'll also benefit from a firsthand look at what the jobs are really like, as told in the words of the employees themselves. Throughout the book, one-on-one interviews with dozens of practicing professionals enrich the text and enhance your understanding of life on the job.

These interviews tell what each job entails, what the duties are, what the lifestyle is like, what the upsides and downsides are. All of the professionals reveal what drew them to the field and how they got started. And to help you make the best career choice for yourself, each professional offers you some expert advice based on years of experience.

Each chapter also lets you see at a glance, with easy-to-reference symbols, the level of education required and salary range for the featured occupations.

So, how do you use this book? Easy. You don't need to run to the library and bury yourself in cumbersome documents from the Bureau of Labor Statistics, nor do you need to rush out and buy a lot of bulky books you'll never plow through. All you have to do is glance through our extensive table of contents, find the fields that interest you, and read what the experts have to say.

Introduction to the Field

People who work in the helping professions give of themselves in many different capacities, providing a valuable service to other people in need. Since you're reading this book, chances are you're already considering a career in one of the many areas of this wide-open occupational category. Glancing through the table of contents will give you an idea of all the choices open to you.

But perhaps you're not sure of the working conditions the different fields offer or which area would suit your personality, skills, and lifestyle the most. There are several factors to consider when deciding which sector to pursue. Each field carries with it different levels of responsibility and commitment. To identify occupations that will match your expectations, you need to know what each job entails.

Ask yourself the following questions and make note of your answers. Then, as you go through the chapters, compare your requirements with the information provided by the professionals interviewed. Their comments will help you pinpoint the fields that would interest you, and eliminate those that would clearly be the wrong choice.

- How much time are you willing to commit to training? Some skills can be learned on-the-job or in a year or two of formal training; others can take considerably longer.

- How much money are you willing or able to invest in that training, or possibly in starting a private practice? For some fields the outlay can be daunting. New graduates can start out owing thousands of dollars.

- How much money do you expect to earn after you graduate and after you have a few years' experience under your belt? In general, those areas that pay the most also require the largest investment of time and money.

- How much patient or client care do you want to be involved in? Not every field offers the same amount or same type of people contact.

- How strong is your interest in the actual science supporting the different fields? Some occupations require more knowledge and more involvement than others.

- Can you handle a certain amount of stress on the job, or would you prefer a quiet—and safe—environment?

- Will you work normal hours? Or will your day start at 5:30 A.M. and not end until 13 or 14 hours later? Can you handle emergency calls in the middle of the night? Do you want your weekends free?

- How much independence do you require? Do you want to be your own boss or will you be content as a salaried employee?

Knowing what your expectations are, then comparing them to the realities of the work will help you make informed choices. Although *On the Job: Real People Working in the Helping Professions* strives to be as comprehensive as possible, not all jobs in this extensive field have been covered here or given the same amount of emphasis. You will find information on other related professions in the following *On the Job* books:

On the Job: Real People Working in Service Businesses
On the Job: Real People Working in Government
On the Job: Real People Working in Health Care

If you still have questions after reading this book, there are a number of other avenues to pursue. You can find out more information by contacting the sources listed at the end of each chapter. You can also find professionals on your own to talk to and observe as they go about their work. Any remaining gaps you discover can be filled by referring to the *Occupational Outlook Handbook*.

CHAPTER 1

Human Services Workers

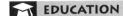
EDUCATION

H.S. Required
Some College Preferred

$$$ SALARY/EARNINGS

$13,000 to $27,000

OVERVIEW

Human services worker is a generic term for people with various job titles, such as social service technician, case management aide, social work assistant, residential counselor, alcohol or drug abuse counselor, mental health technician, child abuse worker, community outreach worker, and gerontology aide.

They generally work under the direction of social workers or, in some cases, psychologists. The amount of responsibility and supervision they are given varies a great deal. Some are on their own most of the time and have little direct supervision; others work under close direction.

Human services workers help clients obtain benefits or services. They assess the needs and establish the eligibility of clients for services. They examine financial documents such as rent receipts and tax returns to determine whether the client is eligible for food stamps, Medicaid, or other welfare programs, for example. They also inform clients how to obtain services; arrange for transportation and escorts, if necessary; and provide emotional support.

Human services workers monitor and keep case records on clients and report progress to supervisors.

Human services workers may transport or accompany clients to group meal sites, adult daycare programs, or doctors' offices; telephone or visit clients' homes to make sure services are being received; or help resolve disagreements, such as those between tenants and landlords.

Human services workers play a variety of roles in community settings. They may organize and lead group activities, assist clients in need of counseling or crisis intervention, or administer a food bank or emergency fuel program.

In halfway houses and group homes, they oversee adult residents who need some supervision or support on a daily basis, but who do not need to live in an institution. They review clients' records, talk with their families, and confer with medical personnel to gain better insight into their background and needs. Human services workers may teach residents to prepare their own meals and to do other housekeeping activities. They also provide emotional support and lead recreation activities.

In mental hospitals and psychiatric clinics, they may help clients master everyday living skills and teach them how to communicate more effectively and get along better with others. They also assist with music, art, and dance therapy and with individual and group counseling and lead recreational activities.

Working conditions of human services workers vary. Many spend part of their time in an office or group residential facility and the rest in the field visiting clients or taking them on trips, or meeting with people who provide services to the clients.

Most work a regular 40-hour week, although some work may be in the evening and on weekends. Human services workers in residential settings generally work in shifts because residents need supervision around the clock.

The work, while satisfying, can be emotionally draining. Understaffing and lack of equipment may add to the pressure. Turnover is reported to be high, especially among workers without academic preparation for this field.

TRAINING

While some employers hire high school graduates, most prefer applicants with some college preparation in human services, social work, or one of the social or behavioral sciences. Some prefer to hire persons with a four-year college degree. The level of formal education of human service workers often influences the kind of work they are assigned and the amount of responsibility entrusted to them. Workers with no more than a high school education are likely to perform clerical duties, while those with a college degree might be assigned to do direct counseling, coordinate program activities, or manage a group home.

Employers may also look for experience in other occupations or leadership experience in school or in a youth group. Some enter the field on the basis of courses in social work, psychology, sociology, rehabilitation, or special education. Most employers provide in-service training such as seminars and workshops.

Because so many human services jobs involve direct contact with people who are vulnerable to exploitation or mistreatment, employers try to select applicants with appropriate personal qualifications. Relevant academic preparation is generally required, and volunteer or work experience is preferred. A strong desire to help others, patience, and understanding are highly valued characteristics. Other important personal traits include communication skills, a strong sense of responsibility, and the ability to manage time effectively. Hiring requirements in group homes tend to be more stringent than in other settings.

In 1994, 375 certificate and associate degree programs in human services or mental health were offered at community and junior colleges, vocational-technical institutes, and other post-secondary institutions. In addition, 390 programs offered a bachelor's degree in human services. A small number of programs leading to master's degrees in human services administration were offered as well.

Generally, academic programs in this field educate students for specialized roles—work with developmentally disabled adults, for example. Students are exposed early and often to the kinds of situations they may encounter on the job. Programs typically include courses in psychology, sociology, crisis intervention, social work, family dynamics, therapeutic interviewing, rehabilitation, and gerontology. Through classroom simulation and internships, students learn interview, observation, and recordkeeping skills; individual and group counseling techniques; and program planning.

Formal education is almost always necessary for advancement. In group homes, completion of a one-year certificate in human services along with several years of experience may suffice for promotion to supervisor. In general, however, advancement requires a bachelor's or master's degree in counseling, rehabilitation, social work, or a related field.

JOB OUTLOOK

Human services workers held about 168,000 jobs in 1994. About one-fourth were employed by state and local governments, primarily in public welfare agencies and facilities for the mentally retarded and developmentally disabled. Another fourth worked in private social services agencies offering a variety of services, including adult daycare, group meals, crisis intervention, and counseling. Still another fourth supervised residents of group homes and halfway houses. Human services workers also held jobs in clinics, community mental health centers, and psychiatric hospitals.

Opportunities for human services workers are expected to be excellent for qualified applicants. The number of human services workers is projected to grow much faster than the average for all occupations between 1994 and the year 2005—ranking among the most rapidly growing occupations.

Also, the need to replace workers who retire or stop working for other reasons will create additional job opportunities. However, these jobs are not attractive to everyone because the work requires responsibility and is emotionally draining and most jobs offer relatively poor pay, so qualified applicants should have little difficulty finding employment.

Opportunities are expected to be best in job training programs, residential settings, and private social service agencies, which include such services as adult daycare and meal delivery programs. Demand for these services will expand with the growing number of older people, who are more likely to need services.

In addition, human services workers will continue to be needed to provide services to the mentally impaired and developmentally disabled, those with substance abuse problems, and a wide variety of others.

Faced with rapid growth in the demand for services, but slower growth in resources to provide the services, employers are expected to rely increasingly on human services workers rather than other occupations that command higher pay.

Job training programs are expected to require additional human services workers as the economy grows and businesses change their mode of production and workers need to be retrained. Human services workers help determine workers' eligibility for public assistance programs and help them obtain services while unemployed.

Residential settings should expand also as pressures to respond to the needs of the chronically mentally ill persist. For many years, chronic mental patients have been deinstitutionalized and left to their own devices. Now, more community-based programs and group residences are expected to be established to house and assist the homeless and chronically mentally ill, and demand for human services workers will increase accordingly.

Although overall employment in state and local governments will grow only as fast as the average for all industries, jobs for human services workers will grow more rapidly. State and local governments employ most of their human services workers in correctional and public assistance departments. Correctional departments are growing faster than other areas of government, so human services workers should find their job opportunities increase along with other corrections jobs. Public assistance programs have been relatively stable within governments' budgets, but they have been employing more human services workers in an attempt to employ fewer social workers, who are more educated and higher paid.

SALARIES

According to limited data available, starting salaries for human services workers ranged from about $13,000 to $20,000 a year in 1994. Experienced workers generally earned between $18,000 and $27,000 annually, depending on their education, experience, and employer.

RELATED FIELDS

Workers in other occupations that require skills similar to those of human services workers include social workers, community outreach workers, religious workers, occupational therapy assistants, physical therapy assistants and aides, psychiatric aides, and activity leaders.

∎INTERVIEW

M. Allen Broyles
Residential Counselor

M. Allen Broyles has worked in a group home for the mentally impaired since 1992. He is responsible for teaching independent living skills to the residents.

What the Job's Really Like

"Jadwin House, the group home I work in, is owned by Sunderland Family Treatment Services, an outpatient counseling service organization for the community. It houses up to eight residents who have been released from mental institutions and want to learn how to live on their own.

"I teach the residents independent living skills. This includes personal hygiene, money management, time management, cooking skills, etc. All the skills and tools each individual may need to live on his or her own.

"These are 'hands on' applications. Most of my teaching is how to cook and how to do their daily housecleaning chores. I show them cooking procedures such as how to use cutlery or follow recipes. I also help teach them about budgeting, time management and work habits.

"I work the swing shift—the busiest shift of the day. I am the only staff member on duty from 3:00 P.M. to 11:00 P.M. I get to work, then take a few minutes briefing from the day shift as to any unusual developments during the day—new residents, new procedures, medicine changes, that sort of thing. Most of the residents will be gone at that time, tending to their daily routines. Most of them go to another facility called Wilson House, a day facility that trains our people in working skills. Others are keeping doctor's appointments.

"I make all changes needed at that time in meds and procedures. I may go around and let the residents who are in the house know that I am on duty for their peace of mind. I then check the evening meal sheet to see which resident is assigned cooking duty that evening. Sometimes that resident will be on leave or absent for some reason and I must make alternative plans.

"At around 4:30 P.M. I round up the assigned cook and we start the evening meal. All items on the menu are brought from the food storage area and the resident is brought up to speed on what is going to be prepared. The resident decides what he or she is going to do in preparation. I then show the resident all the things he or she needs to know to accomplish the tasks. I perform the remainder of the cooking to finish the meal. It is my feeling that these residents have very few pleasures in their lives. The evening meal should be one of them. I make every effort to see that they get a pleasurable dinner each day. The resident sets the table and serves the meal home style. This allows the residents to interact with each other at meal time compared to cafeteria style. I like them asking each other to pass the bread, beans, and bouillabaisse.

"After dinner the cook cleans the kitchen and the other residents are assigned other cleaning chores. I see that those chores are accomplished and give instructions when they are needed.

"At 8:00 P.M. I monitor the medications for the evening. Once this is done the residents settle into the evening routines such as watching TV, listening to the stereo, or going for walks. This is a fairly quiet time—except when I pull a fire drill.

"From 9:00 to 11:00 is usually quiet. That is when I get my paperwork done and personal things such as working on my own writing. Sometimes I go out and watch TV with the residents.

"At 11:00 P.M. my relief arrives. I give him a brief on the house and then go home.

"I like being able to help people with their second, third, fourth chances in life. We have seen some very dramatic turn arounds. For example, when Henry came to us he was disheveled and haggard looking. His schizophrenia had him so delusional he was impossible to talk to. Paranoia gripped him so tightly he was afraid to leave the home.

"Henry was with us for three years. He gradually improved and today has his own apartment where he lives alone. He is not working as yet, but the improvements in his quality of life have been dramatic.

"Joanie came to us so paranoid she isolated herself in her room and only came out to eat. There were times we felt she might have to return to the hospital. Today she still hears voices from time to time and her paranoia is still present, but she has learned to control both of them and live on her own. She is now working and being a productive citizen.

"But I don't like the feeling of hopelessness you get when some residents have to be readmitted to the hospital."

How M. Allen Broyles Got Started

"In 1991 I attempted to open a group home for teen boys in this community. My wife and I had been doing teen girls foster care for about ten years for the state of Washington and we saw a huge need for a boys' home. In the effort to start the group home I formed a nonprofit corporation. In selecting board members for the corporation, I had selected the owner of Sunderland. When the finances failed to materialize for the boys' home she offered me my present position. That was in 1992.

"I started college at age 26 after dropping out of high school at the end of my sophomore year. By the time I started again I had a wife and two kids. I worked swing shift at Boeing in Seattle and went to school from 8:00 in the morning until 2:00 in the afternoon. This went on for three years. It got to the point my kid hardly knew me. I was so busy getting my 3.5 GPA that it became a matter of my family or my schooling. My family came first. But if I had it to do over again I would not have quit."

Expert Advice

"The main criterion is to be a person who interacts with others well. Do you want to have an impact on people's lives—sometimes at great cost? Are you willing to put up with all the downsides of mental illness to see the positive effects later? Do you really care about the well-being of those less fortunate than yourself?

"This field is taking on some major changes. With government pulling in the purse strings, this field is downsizing. We are now more results-oriented than maintenance-oriented. Our tracking of the care we give needs to show how the patient is improving and moving toward the goal of self-sufficiency. It used to be that we could work slower for our results than we can today. Now we have alternative goals that move the resident on quicker.

"My last suggestion is that you educate yourself as far as possible. The higher your education and the more specialized that education is, the more successful you will find yourself with these new changes."

●　　●　　●

FOR MORE INFORMATION

Information on academic programs in human services may be found in most directories of two- and four-year colleges, available at libraries or career counseling centers.

For information on programs and careers in human services, contact:

National Organization for Human Service Education
Brookdale Community College
Lyncroft, NJ 07738

Council for Standards in Human Service Education
Montgomery Community College
340 Dekalb Pike
Blue Bell, PA 19422

Information on job openings may be available from state employment service offices or directly from city, county, or state departments of health, mental health and mental retardation, and human resources.

CHAPTER 2 Social Workers

EDUCATION

B.A./B.S. Required
Postgraduate Preferred

$$$ SALARY/EARNINGS

$17,500 to $44,000

OVERVIEW

Social workers help people. They help individuals cope with problems such as inadequate housing, unemployment, lack of job skills, financial mismanagement, serious illness, disability, substance abuse, unwanted pregnancy, or antisocial behavior. They also work with families that have serious conflicts, including those involving child or spousal abuse.

Through direct counseling, social workers help clients identify their real concerns and help them to consider solutions and find resources. Often, social workers provide concrete information such as where to go for debt counseling; how to find child care or elder care; how to apply for public assistance or other benefits; or how to get an alcoholic or drug addict admitted to a rehabilitation program.

Social workers may also arrange for services in consultation with clients and then follow through to ensure the services are actually helpful. They may review eligibility requirements, fill out forms and applications, arrange for services, visit clients on a regular basis, and step in during emergencies.

Most social workers specialize in a clinical field such as child welfare and family services, mental health, medical social work, or school social work.

CLINICAL SOCIAL WORKERS offer psychotherapy or counseling and a range of services in public agencies and clinics as well as in private practice. Other social workers are employed in community organization, administration, or research.

SOCIAL WORKERS IN CHILD WELFARE OR FAMILY SERVICES may counsel children and youths who have difficulty adjusting socially, advise parents on how to care for disabled children, or arrange for homemaker services during a parent's illness. If children have serious problems in school, child welfare workers may consult with parents, teachers, and counselors to identify underlying causes and develop plans for treatment.

Some social workers assist single parents, arrange adoptions, and help find foster homes for neglected or abandoned children. Child welfare workers also work in residential institutions for children and adolescents.

Social workers in child or adult protective services investigate reports of abuse and neglect and intervene if necessary. They may institute legal action to remove children from homes and place them temporarily in an emergency shelter or with a foster family.

MENTAL HEALTH SOCIAL WORKERS provide services for persons with mental or emotional problems, such as individual and group therapy, outreach, crisis intervention, social rehabilitation, and training in skills of everyday living. They may also help plan for supportive services to ease patients' return to the community.

MEDICAL SOCIAL WORKERS help patients and their families cope with chronic, acute, or terminal illnesses and handle problems that may stand in the way of recovery or rehabilitation. They may organize support groups for families of patients suffering from cancer, AIDS, Alzheimer's disease, or other illnesses. They also advise family caregivers, and counsel patients and help plan for their needs after discharge by arranging for at-home services from meals-on-wheels to oxygen equipment. Some work on interdisciplinary teams that evaluate certain kinds of patients—geriatric or transplant patients, for example.

SCHOOL SOCIAL WORKERS diagnose students' problems and arrange needed services, counsel children in trouble, and help integrate disabled students into the general school population. School social workers deal with problems such as student pregnancy, misbehavior in class, and excessive absences. They also advise teachers on how to deal with problem students.

SOCIAL WORKERS IN CRIMINAL JUSTICE make recommendations to courts, do pre-sentencing assessments, and provide services for prison inmates and their families. Probation and parole officers provide similar services to individuals on parole or sentenced by a court to probation.

INDUSTRIAL OR OCCUPATIONAL SOCIAL WORKERS generally work in an employer's personnel department or health unit. Through employee assistance programs, they help workers cope with job-related pressures or personal problems that affect the quality of their work. They offer direct counseling to employees, often those whose performance is hindered by emotional or family problems or substance abuse. They also develop education programs and refer workers to specialized community programs.

SOCIAL WORKERS SPECIALIZING IN GERONTOLOGICAL SERVICES run support groups for family caregivers or for the adult children of aging parents; advise elderly people or family members about the choices in such areas as housing, transportation, and long-term care; and coordinate and monitor services.

Most social workers have a standard 40-hour week. However, they may work some evenings and weekends to meet with clients, attend community meetings, and handle emergencies. Some, particularly in voluntary nonprofit agencies, work part time.

They may spend most of their time in an office or residential facility, but may also travel locally to visit clients or meet with service providers.

The work, while satisfying, can be emotionally draining. Understaffing and large caseloads add to the pressure in some agencies.

TRAINING

A bachelor's degree is the minimum requirement for most positions. Besides the bachelor's in social work (B.S.W.), undergraduate majors in psychology, sociology, and related fields satisfy hiring requirements in some agencies, especially small community agencies.

A master's degree in social work (M.S.W.) is generally necessary for positions in health and mental health settings. Jobs in public agencies may also require an M.S.W. Supervisory, administrative, and staff training positions usually require at least an M.S.W. College and university teaching positions and most research appointments normally require a doctorate in social work.

In 1994, the Council on Social Work Education accredited 383 B.S.W. programs and 117 M.S.W. programs. There were 56 doctoral programs for Ph.D.s in social work and D.S.W.s (Doctor of Social Work).

B.S.W. programs prepare graduates for direct service positions such as caseworker or group worker. They include courses in social work practice, social welfare policies, human behavior and the social environment, and social research methods. Accredited B.S.W. programs require at least 400 hours of supervised field experience.

An M.S.W. degree prepares graduates to perform assessments, to manage cases, and to supervise other workers. Master's programs usually last two years and include 900 hours of supervised field instruction, or internship. Entry into an M.S.W. program does not require a bachelor's in social work, but courses in psychology, biology, sociology, economics, political science, history, social anthropology, urban studies, and social work are recommended. Some schools offer an accelerated M.S.W program for those with a B.S.W.

Social workers may advance to supervisor, program manager, assistant director, and finally to executive director of an agency or department. Advancement generally requires an M.S.W., as well as experience. Other career options for social workers are teaching, research, and consulting. Some help formulate government policies by analyzing and advocating policy positions in government agencies, in research institutions, and on legislators' staffs.

Some social workers go into private practice. Most private practitioners are clinical social workers who provide psychotherapeutic counseling, usually paid through health insurance. Private practitioners must have completed an M.S.W. and a period of supervised work experience. A network of contacts for referrals is also essential.

Since 1993, all states and the District of Columbia had licensing, certification, or registration laws regarding social work practice and the use of professional titles. In addition, voluntary certification is offered by the National Association of Social Workers (NASW), which grants the titled ACSW (Academy of Certified Social Workers) or ACBSW (Academy of Certified Baccalaureate Social Workers) to those who qualify. For clinical social workers, professional credentials include listing in the NASW Register of Clinical Social Workers or in the Directory of American Board of Examiners in Clinical Social Work. These credentials are particularly important for those in private practice; some health insurance providers require them for reimbursement.

JOB OUTLOOK

Social workers held about 557,000 jobs in 1994. Nearly 40 percent of the jobs were in state, county, or municipal government agencies, primarily in departments of human resources, social services, child welfare, mental health, health, housing, education, and corrections.

Most in the private sector were in voluntary social service agencies, community and religious organizations, hospitals, nursing homes, or home health agencies.

Although most social workers are employed in cities or suburbs, some work in rural areas.

Employment of social workers is expected to increase faster than the average for all occupations through the year 2005. The number of older people, who are more likely to need social services, is growing rapidly. In addition, requirements for social workers will grow with increases in the need for and concern about services to the mentally ill, the mentally retarded, and individuals and families in crisis. Many job openings will also arise due to the need to replace social workers who leave the occupation.

Employment of social workers in hospitals is projected to grow much faster than the average for the economy as a whole due to greater emphasis on discharge planning, which facilitates early discharge of patients by assuring that the necessary medical services and social supports are in place when individuals leave the hospital.

Employment of social workers in private social service agencies will grow, but not as rapidly as demand for their services. Agencies will increasingly restructure services and hire more lower-paid human services workers instead of social workers.

Employment in government should also grow in response to increasing needs for public welfare and family services. However, employment levels will depend on government funding for various social service programs.

Social worker employment in home health care services is growing, not only because hospitals are moving to release patients more quickly, but because a large and growing number of people have impairments or disabilities that make it difficult to live at home without some form of assistance.

Opportunities for social workers in private practice will expand because of the anticipated availability of funding from health insurance and from public sector contracts. Also, with increasing affluence, people will be more willing to pay for professional help to deal with personal problems. The growing popularity of employee assistance programs is also expected to spur demand for private practitioners, some of whom provide social work services to corporations on a contract basis.

Employment of school social workers is expected to grow, due to expanded efforts to respond to the adjustment problems of immigrants, children from single-parent families, and others in difficult situations. Moreover, continued emphasis on integrating disabled children into the general school population—a requirement under the Education for All Handicapped Children Act—will probably lead to more jobs. The availability of state and local funding will dictate the actual increase in jobs in this setting, however.

Competition for social worker jobs is stronger in cities, where training programs for social workers abound; rural areas often find it difficult to attract and retain qualified staff.

SALARIES

According to a membership survey of the National Association of Social Workers, social workers with M.S.W. degrees had median earnings of $30,000 in 1993. For those with B.S.W. degrees, median earnings were between $17,500 and $20,000 according to the same survey.

In hospitals, social workers who worked full-time averaged about $33,300 in 1994, according to a survey performed by the University of Texas Medical Branch. Salaries ranged from a minimum of about $26,700 to a maximum of about $40,100.

Social workers employed by the federal government averaged $44,000 in 1995.

RELATED FIELDS

Through direct counseling or referral to other services, social workers help people solve a range of personal problems. Workers in occupations with similar duties include the clergy, counselors, counseling and clinical psychologists, psychotherapists, and vocational rehabilitation counselors.

INTERVIEW
Patricia Morin
Clinical Social Worker

Patricia Morin has a private practice in Grand View, New York. She earned her B.A. in psychology at Fairfield University in Connecticut; her M.A. in counseling psychology, also at Fairfield University; and her M.S.W. at Hunter College in New York City. She also earned a C.S.W., a New York State certification that allows for third-party payments for services. She has been working in the field since 1974.

What the Job's Really Like

"I see individuals who are depressed or anxious. They are adults from 18 to 65 and my case load right now is split down the middle—men and women. Two come twice a week, the rest except for one person come once a week (for 50 minutes), and one is terminating and comes once every two weeks but will be moving to once a month.

"Because I deal with so many individuals, an average of 21 to 28, each day is vastly different. What I love most about the job, besides helping individuals, is that I feel free. There is no structure except that which I set for myself. I could see two people in the morning from 9:00 to 11:00, go shopping and do errands, come back at 2:00. Generally, the evening hours are full first because of others' work schedules. I work three evenings from 4:00 to 8:00, three mornings from 9:00 to 11:00.

"The work in this field is intense. In other jobs, you come in to a set place, go to a set area, get a cup of coffee or juice, say hello to people. The average day in that type of setting has maybe five hours maximum of intense work. There are lunch hours and breaks and mind wanderings. As a therapist, you are on from the moment you greet your first appointment. No wanderings, no interruptions are allowed. Some days I see seven people. I am one tired puppy when I am done. But my day is spread out over 12 hours.

"The diversity of people I see is wonderful. The quality of the conversation is unbeatable. I'm not one for too much small talk. I love the depth of the work and meeting all the different types of people. I learn so much from them, also.

"In the work arena, the clients I see share all of what they do and feel. I've learned about carpentry, police work, teaching, what's new in the medical field. People also teach me about what's going on in life, in general.

"There's a lot of paper work. Insurance companies are difficult to work with. HMOs are infiltrating the field and now you have to try to join one so your clients can be covered. They pay a certain amount and that's it. My fee is $75 an hour, some pay $25 of it. Some people cannot afford the other $50. One has to negotiate. Different insurance companies demand different types of paper work and pay different amounts. Most, however, still pay 50 to 80 percent.

"One major problem in private practice is if you have your own family to take care of it's hard. You're always on duty. You like to think that you're not, but it's like wearing a constant beeper without owning one.

"The holidays are very hard for people and I find that's when I am the busiest. I get double the calls and I have to make extra sessions available. It's a truly hectic, tiring, demanding time.

"Let me tell you the worst experience I had in the sheltered workshop I was working in. A woman, 22 (with a 2-year-old), living on her own through Medicaid and welfare, was very agitated. I got called through the intercom that she was in the foyer screaming my name. The secretary asked if she should let her in. I said *no*! She was behind a glass front door (some protection) and I went out to her.

"She had a lead pipe in one hand and a brick in the other. She dared me to come outside. I told her I would if she dropped one of the weapons. If not, I would call the police, she goes to jail, her kid in a home, and I go back to my office. She decided to drop the brick. I wanted her to drop the lead pipe. I walked outside with her and had another counselor at the door covering me. After an hour, she dropped the pipe. It was a three-hour ordeal before I could get to the root of the problem. Her boyfriend had broken up with her. It was a hard population to work with there. I really liked her, though, and I knew she knew it. The power of the negotiation was in the relationship.

"I believe that my main responsibility as a therapist is to set a positive atmosphere so that people can identify and resolve issues (and feelings surrounding those issues) within the stated psychological ethical guidelines. I achieve this through individual, family, or couple therapy.

"After each session, which is usually 45 to 50 minutes for adults and 15 minutes to a half hour for children (ages 5 to 11), I keep notes of the visit. I make sure they are general with little cues for me what the session was about. It's helpful to jot down one or two sentences about what surrounding feelings the client is going through.

"The rewards, intrinsically, are great. The natural high in having someone feel internal peace and self-love is irreplaceable. I got a letter from someone I saw six years ago. He shared how much he learned and how it helped him get through a very difficult situation. He had to write me, he thanked me. There is no greater joy."

How Patricia Morin Got Started

"I was a biochemistry major and was going to study dolphins and sharks. I was going to live on the *Calypso* with Cousteau and teach dolphins sign language. But I couldn't cut a frog or a pig or a cat. I named them all and then I had to bury them. I did not do well in lab.

"While this was going on and I thought of switching my major to English so that I could write about the ocean, girls on the same floor in my dorm would come and talk to me about their problems. The school psychologist suggested that I look into psychology since two of his patients were talking to me on a regular basis and I was a terrific cotherapist. After I got over my initial "shrinks need shrinks" attitude, I took a class, loved the class, but did not do well. It was a total switch from what I was used to in chemistry and microbiology. The psychologist suggested that I take another course and not get disheartened. I took abnormal psychology, a requirement, and I loved it. And I did very well. I fell more in love with learning about human nature in depth and continued on this path to this day.

"My first job was through the university at Fairfield Community Services dealing with drug-involved youth and their families through individual, group, and family counseling under the supervision of a psychiatrist and psychologist. I started as a volunteer, then junior counselor and worked there from 1974 through 1978.

"From 1978 through 1985 I worked at Clarkstown Counseling Center doing the same kind of work. In Clarkstown, I became a senior counselor and an assistant director.

"I left and for a year became a director of a dual diagnosis (mental retardation and schizophrenia) clinic, which was also a sheltered workshop. In this workshop, clients worked a full eight hours and got paid. The jobs were delivered by companies that wanted cheap labor. The clients received a lot of satisfaction and were also often in group homes. The relationships they formed at work helped them eventually get jobs outside of the workshop and in the community. The clinic helped them with relationships on all levels.

"I started my private practice in my home office in 1984.

"The reason that I went from a counseling psych masters to an M.S.W. (in 1982) is I believe in the philosophy and psychology of social work—dealing with the environment, family, and the individual. This also takes into account culture and religion. In counseling, I learned more about testing and the nature of the individual. This was not enough for me. I liked being able to get involved in dream work and the subconscious material. Counseling, at the masters level, did not teach me this. Plus, I found that most agencies wanted their staff to have the M.S.W."

Expert Advice

"First, evaluate what your personal life's philosophy is. If you believe strongest that an individual has the power to change his environment, be a psychologist. If you believe that the individual cannot change his environment, and that the environment has to be worked also, be a clinical social worker. Explore your beliefs about human nature, human values, your values.

"Second, go into therapy. If you haven't gone through it you can't expect others to go through it with you. It's an incredible experience that will help you learn in every way.

"Third, start in a clinic, with a poorer population. They need the help, you need the experience. Although it is low-paying and tough work, you need to pay your dues in this field. The advantage is that you get a taste of every type of diagnosis, every type of person. This will lead you to number four.

"Know what type of client you shouldn't be working with. Don't delude yourself into believing you can see them all. You can't. You're human. I see individuals who are depressed and anxious. I cannot see people who are, for example, diagnosed as histrionic. So I don't see them and they are better off, so am I.

"Last but not least, keep good notes and document client progress or lack of progress."

● ● ●

FOR MORE INFORMATION

For information about career opportunities in social work, contact:

National Association of Social Workers
750 First Street NE, Suite 700
Washington, DC 20002-4241

National Network for Social Work Managers, Inc.
6501 North Federal Highway, Suite 5
Boca Raton, FL 33487

An annual Directory of Accredited B.S.W. and M.S.W. Programs
is available for $10 from:

Council on Social Work Education
1600 Duke Street
Alexandria, VA 22314-3421

3

Mental Health and Rehabilitation Counselors

EDUCATION

Postgraduate Required

$$$ SALARY/EARNINGS

$20,000 to $50,000

OVERVIEW

Counselors assist people with personal, family, social, educational, and career decisions, problems, and concerns. Their duties depend on the individuals they serve and the settings in which they work.

MENTAL HEALTH COUNSELORS emphasize prevention and work with individuals and groups to promote optimum mental health. They help individuals deal with addictions and substance abuse, family, parenting, and marital problems, suicide, stress management, problems with self-esteem, issues associated with aging, job and career concerns, educational decisions, and issues of mental and emotional health.

Mental health counselors work closely with other mental health specialists, including psychiatrists, psychologists, clinical social workers, psychiatric nurses, and school counselors.

Some counselors specialize in a particular social issue or population group, such as marriage and family, grief, multicultural, and gerontological counseling. A gerontological counselor may provide services to elderly persons who face changing lifestyles due to health problems, as well as help families cope with these changes. A multicultural counselor might help employers adjust to an increasingly diverse workforce.

REHABILITATION COUNSELORS help persons deal with the personal, social, and vocational impact of their disabilities. They evaluate the strengths and limitations of individuals, provide personal and vocational counseling, and may arrange for medical care, vocational training, and job placement. Rehabilitation counselors interview individuals with disabilities and their families, evaluate school and medical reports, and confer and plan with physicians, psychologists, occupational therapists, employers, and others. Conferring with the client, they develop and implement a rehabilitation program, which may include training to help the person become more independent and employable. They also work toward increasing the client's capacity to adjust and live independently.

Self-employed counselors and those working in mental health and community agencies often work evenings to counsel clients who work during the day.

Rehabilitation counselors generally work a standard 40-hour week.

Counselors work in a wide variety of public and private establishments. These include health care facilities; vocational rehabilitation centers; social agencies; correctional institutions; and residential care facilities, such as halfway houses for criminal offenders and group homes for children, the aged, and the disabled.

Counselors also worked in organizations engaged in community improvement and social change, as well as drug and alcohol rehabilitation programs and state and local government agencies. A growing number of counselors work in health maintenance organizations, insurance companies, group practice, and private practice, spurred by laws allowing counselors to receive payments from insurance companies, and requiring employers to provide rehabilitation services to injured workers.

TRAINING

Generally, counselors have a master's degree in mental health counseling, counseling psychology, gerontological counseling, marriage and family counseling, substance abuse counseling, rehabilitation counseling, agency or community counseling, or a related field.

Graduate level counselor education programs in colleges and universities usually are in departments of education or psychology. Courses are grouped into eight core areas:

Human growth and development

Social and cultural foundations

Helping relationships

Groups

Lifestyle and career development

Appraisal

Research and evaluation

Professional orientation

In an accredited program, 48 to 60 semester hours of graduate study, including a period of supervised clinical experience in counseling, are required for a master's degree. The Council for Accreditation of Counseling and Related Educational Programs (CACREP) accredits graduate counseling programs in counselor education, and in community, gerontological, mental health, school, student affairs, and marriage and family counseling.

In 1993, 39 states and the District of Columbia had some form of counselor credentialing legislation, licensure, certification, or registry for practice outside schools. Requirements vary from state to state. In some states, credentialing is mandatory; in others, voluntary.

Many counselors elect to be nationally certified by the National Board for Certified Counselors (NBCC), which grants the general practice credential National Certified Counselor. In order to be certified, a counselor must hold a master's degree in counseling, have at least two years of professional counseling experience, and pass NBCC's National Counselor Examination. This national certification is voluntary and distinct from state certification. However, in some states those who pass the national exam are exempt from taking a state certification exam. NBCC also offers specialty certification in career, gerontological, school, and clinical mental health counseling.

Mental health counselors generally have a master's degree in mental health counseling, another area of counseling, or in psychology or social work. They are voluntarily certified by the

National Board of Certified Clinical Mental Health Counselors. Generally, to receive this certification as a mental health counselor, a counselor must have a master's degree in counseling, two years of post-master's experience, a period of supervised clinical experience, a taped sample of clinical work, and a passing grade on a written examination.

Vocational and related rehabilitation agencies generally require a master's degree in rehabilitation counseling, counseling and guidance, or counseling psychology for rehabilitation counselor jobs. Some, however, may accept applicants with a bachelor's degree in rehabilitation services, counseling, psychology, or related fields.

A bachelor's degree in counseling qualifies a person to work as a counseling aide, rehabilitation aide, or social service worker. Experience in employment counseling, job development, psychology, education, or social work may be helpful.

The Council on Rehabilitation Education (CORE) accredits graduate programs in rehabilitation counseling. A minimum of two years of study including a period of supervised clinical experience is required for the master's degree. Some colleges and universities offer a bachelor's degree in rehabilitation services education.

In most state vocational rehabilitation agencies, applicants must pass a written examination and be evaluated by a board of examiners. Many employers require rehabilitation counselors to be certified. To become certified by the Commission on Rehabilitation Counselor Certification, counselors must graduate from an accredited educational program, complete an internship, and pass a written examination. They are then designated as Certified Rehabilitation Counselors.

Some employers provide training for newly hired counselors. Many have work-study programs so that employed counselors can earn graduate degrees. Counselors must participate in graduate studies, workshops, institutes, and personal studies to maintain their certificates and licenses.

Persons interested in counseling should have a strong interest in helping others and the ability to inspire respect, trust, and confidence. They should be able to work independently or as part of a team.

Mental health and rehabilitation counselors may become supervisors or administrators in their agencies. Some counselors move into research, consulting, or college teaching, or go into private practice.

JOB OUTLOOK

Counselors held about 165,000 jobs in 1994. About 7 out of 10 were school counselors. (See Chapter 4 for more information on academic and career counselors.)

Overall employment of counselors is expected to grow faster than the average for all occupations through the year 2005. In addition, replacement needs should increase significantly by the end of the decade as a large number of counselors reach retirement age.

Mental health and rehabilitation counselors should be in strong demand. Insurance companies increasingly provide for reimbursement of counselors, enabling many counselors to move from schools and government agencies to private practice. The number of people who need rehabilitation services will rise as advances in medical technology continue to save lives that only a few years ago would have been lost.

In addition, legislation requiring equal employment rights for persons with disabilities will spur demand for counselors. Counselors not only will help individuals with disabilities with their transition into the workforce, but also will help companies comply with the law.

More mental health and rehabilitation counselors also will be needed as the elderly population grows, and as society focuses on ways of developing mental well-being, such as controlling stress associated with job and family responsibilities.

Similar to other government jobs, the number of employment counselors, who work primarily for state and local governments, could be limited by budgetary constraints.

SALARIES

Self-employed counselors who have well-established practices generally have the highest earnings, as do some counselors working for private companies, such as insurance companies and private rehabilitation companies.

Median earnings for full-time counselors were about $36,100 a year in 1994. The middle 50 percent earned between $26,500 and $46,200 a year. The bottom 10 percent earned less than $20,000 a year, while the top 10 percent earned over $50,000 a year.

RELATED FIELDS

Counselors help people evaluate their interests, abilities, and disabilities, and deal with personal, social, academic, and career problems. Others who help people in similar ways include college and student personnel workers, teachers, personnel workers and managers, human services workers, social workers, psychologists, psychiatrists, members of the clergy, occupational therapists, training and employee development specialists, and equal employment opportunity/affirmative action specialists.

INTERVIEW

Romney Latko
Marriage, Family, and Child Counselor Trainee

Romney Latko earned her B.A. in psychology in 1994 from San Diego State University. She finished her master's in counseling psychology at the University for Humanistic Studies in Solana Beach, California, and is just starting work on her Ph.D. in clinical psychology at Pacific Graduate School of Psychology, in Palo Alto, California. She expects to graduate in June 1999.

What the Job's Really Like

"I work for New Alternatives Incorporation—Home Based Services. It's a nonprofit organization that holds a contract with the San Diego county to provide 'in-home skills building'—i.e., learning how to handle conflicts, goal setting, decision making, communication, discipline techniques. Our services are free of charge to the clients and we go to their houses.

"My job is really an unpaid internship. I needed 200 hours of face-to-face contact with clients and it has taken me six months to accomplish this.

"My clients are families from every economic class, race, and age. Many of them are referred to us by Child Protective Services. These cases are usually given to counselors that have more experience. I primarily have cases that are self-referred.

"We see them in their homes because many of our clients don't have transportation. Or they have many other excuses not to follow through with court-ordered counseling. We sidestep their excuses and simply meet them in their houses.

"I help my clients with whatever issues are most pressing for them. These include everything from teaching them discipline techniques to helping them learn healthy ways of communication. But we are mostly concerned with helping them set up a support system that they can use whenever they come across another crisis.

"Providing in-home services has been a wonderful way for me to start off in this field. In most counseling situations, clients come into the office and whatever they are discussing—their family, home, etc.—are never actually seen by the counselor. By going to their houses I am able to see the environment in which they live and can meet and work with the entire family. This really gives me a lot of insight into what they are going through in their everyday lives. It also forms a type of connection between the counselor and client that often doesn't happen when the interaction is solely in the office.

"The downside to this is the safety factor. I do not know what type of environment I will be walking into and what type of clients I will be working with. Yes, I have been told that if the situation doesn't 'feel right' to just leave, but there is still the issue of my safety.

"Also, driving all over trying to make it to appointments on time is stressful. For instance, I was caught in a traffic jam today that made me 20 minutes late for the appointment. But what can you do? My job is very interesting. All of my clients' situations have been completely different and it has been a challenge to find the right community resources for each. I have only worked four hours a week with clients, four hours a week with children's groups (where we engage the children in activities to help improve their self-esteem) and three hours of both group and individual supervision (where we are able to present cases that are particularly challenging for us in order to get feedback and help).

"But overall it has been a wonderful experience. It is rare for counselors to have the opportunity to see the environments in which their clients live and because of the constant change of scenery it never becomes boring. Working with people after studying for so many years has been a real eye-opening experience. Everything changes when it's a real person sitting across from you. It's really an exciting field to be in."

How Romney Latko Got Started

"I love the creative aspect of this profession. I've always been a creative person; I've played the piano for 19 years, I paint, write poetry and novels—so I knew that I wouldn't be happy unless I was working in a field where I could use this side of me.

"To be successful a counselor has to come up with a creative treatment plan, specifically set up for each individual. Sometimes I may use expressive arts therapy where I ask the clients to draw their feelings. There are techniques that include dance, music, or writing. Journaling is a wonderful way to help clients express their feelings when they find that speaking them out loud is too dangerous. A counselor must be creative in his or her approach to working with people. If counselors stick to one theory or set of techniques too rigidly, they'll run across problems that simply cannot be worked with that way.

"Starting out, I was interested in both physics and psychology. So I had the choice between attempting to understand the universe or attempting to understand the human mind. Three years ago, I began cowriting a book with Dr. Timothy Leary. We never finished the project, but I was exposed to the research he did in the 1950s. His work with transactional psychology absolutely fascinated me, and it was this experience that helped me make my decision. With Dr. Leary's encouragement, I went back into psychology and am glad I did. I am always amazed at the complexity of the human mind and how wonderfully exciting this field really is.

"This is my first job actually doing therapy. I worked for almost a year as a Child Care Worker where I worked at a residential group home for abused children. The company that runs the group homes also runs New Alternatives. So when I needed to find an internship placement I contacted the same company because of my work history with them.

"We had a brief training at New Alternatives that lasted about six hours and we went over discipline techniques, child development stages, signs of child abuse, etc.

"Eventually, when I finish my doctorate, I would like to become a professor at a four-year university, while seeing clients and doing research into social issues at the same time."

Expert Advice

"If you are just starting out in this field, I would recommend field work. By going to clients' houses, the counselor is simply placed into their lives. They don't have the opportunity to "make themselves presentable" and "get everything under control" before they make the trip to your office. The counselor enters a situation right in the middle and in the context in which it started.

"But field work also takes everything that is taught about creating a safe environment and the counselor having control of a session and throws it all right out the window. In a client's house, the client has complete control over everything. There are more disruptions—if a friend stops by, the phone rings, or all of the neighborhood children come running through the house— and this can make sessions unproductive at times.

"As a trainee, the most important thing to know is to find a good supervisor. Without the help of someone who really knows what he or she is doing, a student can quickly begin to feel extremely overwhelmed and lost. If you begin at a placement and do not feel that you are getting all the help you need in order to feel confident with your work, go to your teachers, your fellow students, past research, or books—anyone or anything who can help you feel comfortable with what you are doing.

"Without guidance the whole experience can become too much to handle."

•   •   •

INTERVIEW

Jane E. Bennett
Vocational Rehabilitation Counselor

Jane E. Bennett works for the Department of Rehabilitative Services for the Commonwealth of Virginia in Fairfax, Virginia. She earned her B.S. in 1984 in Leisure Studies and Services, Therapeutic Recreation from Old Dominion University in Norfolk, Virginia. In 1990 she earned her M.A. in Human Resource Development and Rehabilitation Counseling from George Washington University in Washington, DC.

What the Job's Really Like

"I carry a case load of about 130 clients. I provide case management, guidance and counseling, career exploration, training, job search assistance, job placement assistance, employer contact, and education about disabilities to employers. I am responsible for providing services to my clients based on what their needs are in order to return to the workforce. We are an eligibility program in that we follow criteria for determining clients eligible for services. The criteria are these: (1) must have documentation of a disability; (2) this disability must pose a barrier to employment; (3) the client needs DRS to go back to work; and (4) the client is stable physically and mentally to benefit from the services.

"If he or she is found eligible for services, then the client and I develop what is called an Individual Written Rehabilitation Plan. This plan includes the steps the client must take in order to return to the workforce. Therefore, each plan is very specific to the individual and his or her needs for returning to work. Some may need services as simple as guidance and counseling; writing a résumé; learning how to interview and job search. Others may need skills training that takes some time to obtain. The program is very individually based and each client is treated in that manner.

"Rehabilitation counselors can work in the public industry or private industry. Working in the public industry requires a great deal of paperwork. I feel in order to do my job one needs to be a good time manager as well as a good organizer. My job is very busy. Caseloads tend to be rather large, leaving very little room for down time on the job. I use every bit of my eight hours a day to do my job. Sometimes I do work over 40 hours a week, but not often because of the threat of burnout. This is a job that needs to be left at the office once your day is done.

"In a typical day I see four to five clients for one hour apiece and complete field notes and paperwork for each of these clients. The telephone is probably the most important piece of equipment used in my job. If someone doesn't like the telephone—do not go into rehabilitation counseling. I probably get anywhere from 20 to 40 phone calls a day. If I can get the calls just as they are coming in—great. If not, the calls tend to stack up and I find myself trying to return 20-plus phone calls at the end of the day.

That keeps me very busy, but I'm the type of person who wants to stay busy in a job and I don't mind paperwork. Paperwork is one of the reasons that people leave this job.

"My caseload is about 85 percent psychiatrically impaired. I also work with physically impaired, mentally retarded, and learning disabled people. The whole focus of my job is to assist persons with disabilities in returning to the workforce after the onset of a disability, or for them to obtain employment for the first time. We are not just in the business of finding people jobs, but we are in the business of helping people decide on a career and helping them to move in that direction.

"The best part of the job is seeing the clients succeed and improve their lives and watch their self-esteem and self-worth just blossom. A lot of my clients have dealt with failures all their lives and don't feel that success can happen for them. When it does, it's amazing. It doesn't get any better than that."

How Jane E. Bennett Got Started

"Once I was employed by DRS I was sent to a two-week training entitled 'New Counselor Training.' At this training I was taught the process of rehabilitation from intake with the client to closure of the case. Not all state DRS agencies provide this, but it is a requirement for VA counselors and very beneficial.

"I have been through a variety of trainings as a state employee as well, including Americans with Disabilities Act training; working with the deaf and hard of hearing training; computer training; working with difficult clients; working with head-injured clients; rehabilitation technology—just to mention a few. In the three years I have been with DRS I attended about two to three training sessions a year.

"In my careers I have always worked with persons with disabilities, first as a recreation therapist, now as a rehabilitation counselor. When I made the change to rehabilitation counseling, I had decided that I still wanted to continue working with persons with disabilities—but in a counseling role. After quite a bit of research I decided on rehabilitation counseling. I enjoy working with my clients and assisting them to become more independent and increasing their quality of life."

Expert Advice

"For someone wanting to go into rehabilitation counseling, I would say, if you are organized, a good time manager, and enjoy assisting people in increasing their quality of life, then go for it.

"This is a busy, yet very rewarding career. There are times when this job can get overwhelming, but those times are minimized by the success stories. Do not come into this profession looking for an easy job, because it isn't. It is a challenging career that keeps you on your toes."

• • •

FOR MORE INFORMATION

For general information about counseling, as well as information on specialties such as mental health, rehabilitation, multicultural, marriage and family, and gerontological counseling, contact:

> American Counseling Association
> 5999 Stevenson Avenue
> Alexandria, VA 22304

For information on accredited counseling and related training programs, contact:

> Council for Accreditation of Counseling and Related Educational Programs
> American Counseling Association
> 5999 Stevenson Avenue
> Alexandria, VA 22304

For information on national certification requirements and procedures for counselors, contact:

> National Board for Certified Counselors
> 3-D Terrace Way
> Greensboro, NC 27403

For information about rehabilitation counseling, contact:

> National Rehabilitation Counseling Association
> 1910 Association Drive
> Reston, VA 22091

> National Council on Rehabilitation Education
> Department of Special Education
> Utah State University
> Logan, UT 84322-2870

For information on certification requirements for rehabilitation counselors, contact:

> Commission on Rehabilitation Counselor Certification
> 1835 Rohlwing Road, Suite E
> Rolling Meadows, IL 60008

State departments of education can supply information on colleges and universities that offer approved guidance and counseling training for state certification and licensure requirements.

State employment service offices have information about job opportunities and entrance requirements for counselors.

CHAPTER 4 School, College, and Career Counselors

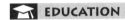 **EDUCATION**

Postgraduate Required

$$$ SALARY/EARNINGS

$20,000 to $50,000

OVERVIEW

SCHOOL AND COLLEGE COUNSELORS help students understand their abilities, interests, talents, and personality characteristics so that the student can develop realistic academic and career options. Counselors use interviews, counseling sessions, tests, or other tools to assist them in evaluating and advising students. They may operate career information centers and career education programs.

HIGH SCHOOL COUNSELORS advise on college majors, admission requirements, entrance exams, and financial aid, and on trade, technical school, and apprenticeship programs. They help students develop job-finding skills such as résumé writing and interviewing techniques.

Counselors also help students understand and deal with their social, behavioral, and personal problems. They emphasize preventive and developmental counseling to provide students with the life skills needed to deal with problems before they occur, and to enhance personal, social, and academic growth. Counselors provide special services, including alcohol and drug prevention programs, and classes that teach students to handle conflicts without resorting to violence.

Counselors work with students individually, in small groups, or with entire classes. Counselors consult and work with parents, teachers, school administrators, school psychologists, school nurses, and social workers.

ELEMENTARY SCHOOL COUNSELORS do more social and personal counseling and less vocational and academic counseling than secondary school counselors. They observe younger children during classroom and play activities and confer with their teachers and parents to evaluate their strengths, problems, or special needs. They also help students develop good study habits.

Most school counselors work the traditional 9- to 10-month school year with a 2- to 3-month vacation, although an increasing number are employed on 10½- or 11-month contracts. They generally have the same hours as teachers.

COLLEGE CAREER PLANNING AND PLACEMENT COUN-SELORS help students and alumni with career development and job hunting. They may assist with writing résumés and improving job interviewing techniques.

EMPLOYMENT COUNSELORS help individuals make wise career decisions. They help clients explore and evaluate their education, training, work history, interests, skills, personal traits, and physical capacities, and may arrange for aptitude and achievement tests. They also work with individuals in developing job-seeking skills and assist clients in locating and applying for jobs.

Counselors work in a wide variety of public and private establishments. These include schools and colleges, job training, career development, and vocational rehabilitation centers; social agencies; and correctional institutions

TRAINING

Generally, counselors have a master's degree in college student affairs, elementary or secondary school counseling, career counseling, or a related field.

All states require school counselors to hold state school counseling certification; however, certification varies from state to state. Some states require public school counselors to have both counseling and teaching certificates.

Depending on the state, a master's degree in counseling and two to five years of teaching experience may be required for a counseling certificate.

Some states require counselors in public employment offices to have a master's degree; others accept a bachelor's degree with appropriate counseling courses.

Prospects for advancement vary by counseling field. School counselors may move to a larger school; become directors or supervisors of counseling or pupil personnel services; or, usually with further graduate education, become counselor educators, counseling psychologists, or school administrators.

Employment counselors may become supervisors or administrators in their agencies.

Some counselors move into research, consulting, or college teaching, or go into private practice.

See Chapter 3 for information on training for all types of counseling professionals.

JOB OUTLOOK

Counselors held about 165,000 jobs in 1994. About 7 out of 10 were school counselors.

Employment of school counselors is expected to grow because of increasing enrollments, particularly in secondary schools, state legislation requiring counselors in elementary schools, and the expanded responsibilities of counselors. Counselors increasingly are becoming involved in crisis and preventive counseling, helping students deal with issues ranging from drug and alcohol abuse to death and suicide. Despite the increasing use of counselors, however, employment growth may be dampened by budgetary constraints. Some counselors serve more than one school.

Employment counselors working in private job training services, however, should grow rapidly as counselors provide skill training and other services to a growing number of laid-off workers, experienced workers seeking a new or second career, full-time homemakers seeking to enter or reenter the work force, and workers who want to upgrade their skills.

SALARIES

Median earnings for full-time educational and vocational counselors were about $36,100 a year in 1994. The middle 50 percent earned between $26,500 and $46,200 a year. The bottom 10 percent earned less than $20,000 a year, while the top 10 percent earned over $50,000 a year.

The average salary of school counselors in the 1994–95 academic year was about $42,500, according to the Educational Research Service. Some school counselors earn additional income working summers in the school system or in other jobs.

RELATED FIELDS

Counselors help people evaluate their interests, abilities, and disabilities, and deal with personal, social, academic, and career problems. Others who help people in similar ways include college and student personnel workers, teachers, personnel workers and managers, human services workers, social workers, psychologists, psychiatrists, members of the clergy, occupational therapists, training and employee development specialists, and equal employment opportunity/affirmative action specialists.

INTERVIEW

Terrence Place
High School Guidance Counselor

Terrence Place is director of the freshman program at Douglas High School in Parkland, Florida. He started his career in 1968 teaching and guidance counseling, then directing guidance programs at a variety of South Florida schools. He has a B.A. in English Education from Florida Southern College in Lakeland and his M.Ed. in counseling from Florida Atlantic University in Boca Raton. He came to his present job at Douglas when the school opened in 1989.

What the Job's Really Like

"I coordinate the orientation and registration of incoming eighth graders from the middle schools, which is really when I pick them up, about halfway through the eighth grade year. As a matter of fact, I'm meeting with about 1,000 parents and students this evening to talk about next year's program, the importance of it and requirements for graduation. We'll also discuss how they shouldn't think that what they're doing is selecting classes for a single year. We want them to realize that they're on the start of a road toward a career.

"We don't like to mention college right away because we want to make sure that the kids understand that it's not just that they'll go to college. In actuality, they'll be going to work some day and that's what they have to plan for.

"We want them to think in terms of careers. For some careers they'd have to go to college, so they'll take a little bit different program, and other kids will have another program. But everyone is going to work, so that's the focus.

"We try to avoid the caste system—that the college kids are better than the kids going to work right after high school. In the past 30 years the percentage of careers requiring college has not changed one percentage point—it's sitting right there between 19 and 20 percent. But the ones that require some sort of post-secondary training, i.e., not college, have risen up to 70 percent from 30 percent. So the skilled labor force is really where all the activity is.

"Once the kids get to Douglas in the ninth grade we spend the first five weeks or so out in classrooms doing a 'let's look where we are today.' Here's what high school grades mean—here's what a high school record looks like and this is what is sent to your employer or college, etc.

"Then, after they get their first set of grades, we start developing a four-year plan. We talk about where they want to be four years from today. Do you want to be college-accepted, moving toward this career, or do you want to be in the armed forces moving toward another career, or in trade or technical school toward yet a different career. The plan is to get them there.

"The plan is reevaluated each year depending on how they did the previous year and what new interests they might have developed. If we put it in stone we'd be throwing away a lot of rocks. What it does do is get the kids to start thinking.

"We tell the kids that they'll be taking seven classes, one of which has to relate to a potential career. Let's say that a kid says to me, 'I'm thinking about something athletic-related,' or he wants to be an athletic trainer. Then we look right away at medical skills, because it's a program that deals with all those types of careers. If a kid said to me he wanted to go into accounting, we might really be looking at business management or law or business computer applications. This way every year they're doing some experimentation. Some of the kids will come in halfway through and say, 'you made me take this class but I hate it.' I say great—now we know what you don't want. And that's a big part of knowing what you do want.

"About 85 percent of our students do go on to college. We start talking to them about different colleges, in state, out of state, large school, small school, do I want to play athletics, etc. What we do is encourage the kids by their junior year to have a list of ten schools they are potentially interested in. We have a county college night, and 300 colleges come and the students can touch base with them then. Or during the summer when they go on a family vacation they can visit the schools then. The purpose of this is so that in their senior year they're all set to apply to five. The five would include a stretch school—that one ideal school, and then at the other end a sure thing and then the in between.

"I'd like to earn a lot more money, of course—and I'd like to work more human hours. I'm here from 6:30 to 4:00. I only get the month of July off.

"But the kids are the best part of my job. Parents—you can keep them all. Good students, bad students, school interested, not school interested. I like them all. This is my 28th year and sometimes I sit on my back porch in the morning having a cup of coffee and I think I just can't face it, I just can't do it. But once I get in to school and talk to the first kid the day goes very quickly."

How Terrence Place Got Started

"I believe personally that 50 percent of career choices are purely accidental. Even with all the guidance. I was a premed major. I got to my junior year and became unsure that was what I really wanted to do. I was thinking about dentistry, too. But my Dad was a teacher and he suggested I take an education course. For part of that requirement I had to spend 60 hours in a classroom. And I fell in love with it.

"I taught for two years, English and social studies, and then they had a guidance position open in my school. At that point, if you already had 15 credits in guidance and counseling, you could become a counselor as long as you signed an agreement that you would finish your master's. So I went ahead with it."

Expert Advice

"I would encourage this career. Certainly education has been tremendously rewarding to me. I believe that teachers are born and not made. I have never seen someone go into a college of education who I didn't think beforehand would be a good teacher and come out a good teacher. I think you possess the personal attributes and they have to be people-centered, being a great listener and truly believing you can make a difference. As far as I'm concerned, I'm a teacher placed in guidance. Everything you do will be to teach a kid something."

● ● ●

INTERVIEW
Cheryl Trull
Adult Education Counselor

Cheryl Trull has worked in her county's Adult Education program for two years counseling GED students. She earned her B.A. in psychology in 1992 and an M.Ed. in counseling in 1994.

What the Job's Really Like

"My office is in the trunk of my car. I travel around to various sites operated by the county's adult education office, counseling students who are studying for their GED. The students range in age from 16 to all the way up. They, for one reason or another, didn't finish their high school education, but now want to take the GED exam.

"The sites are in a variety of places. There's one at the prison, one at a mall; the rest are mainly in churches or community centers. Some are in actual schools, but there the GED program runs at night.

"Each site has at least one GED teacher, if not two, depending on the enrollment. I visit the different centers on a rotating basis, bringing my bag of tricks with me.

"Usually, I try to see each student individually at least once, to discuss their goals for after they pass the GED. I also work with them in small groups. I tell them about various vocational training programs and the different programs the community college offers. I always encourage them to go for some type of training. The more training they have, the better the job they'll be able to get.

"But often, they're not sure what they want to do, what kind of job would suit them. I try to help them to define their interests and to see how that might match up with their skills and how much time they're willing to put in for further training. We do some values clarification and sometimes I work with interest inventories. This helps to narrow down the possibilities.

"A few times a year I also administer the GED exam. That involves about four days of sitting there while students take the exam. It's busy at first, when you're signing everyone in and explaining the rules, but then it gets boring. I always bring a book with me.

"I work 30 hours a week, sometimes less—that depends upon the director and the enrollment figures. It's a good hourly wage, but it's still considered part-time and there are no benefits attached, no sick leave or health insurance.

"The driving aspect makes the job less than desirable for me. There's the traffic, and then my car is always filled up with papers and books and office supplies. I'd much rather have my own permanent office.

"The rewards come from learning that your students passed the exam and went on for more training and then into a good job. That can be very fulfilling, knowing you've helped someone with his or her future."

How Cheryl Trull Got Started

"My original goal was to be a psychologist and have a private practice. While I was getting my master's I did an internship in the counseling center at my university and I enjoyed that very much. But after I graduated I got a job in a mental health unit in a hospital, and then found out that the work didn't really appeal to me—at least not in that setting.

"I took the Adult Ed job as a stop-gap, while I decided what I really want to do. Because the county won't offer any job security or benefits, I won't be able to stay with this job forever. I've been accepted into a Psy.D. program in counseling psychology and I'm going to start my studies next fall. My ultimate goal is to work full-time in a college counseling center and to have a part-time private practice. At least through the different settings I've worked in, I've learned what appeals to me and what doesn't."

Expert Advice

"Finding your own niche is very important. You might have a fantasy about what a job would be like, but you really won't know much about it—if it would suit you or not—until you have first-hand experience. My suggestion is to try to get a variety of internships while you're going for your master's degree. And if you can do it at the bachelor's level, even better. A lot of schools have cooperative education programs. It takes a little longer to get your degree that way, but during the semesters you're working, you can be placed in different settings so you can get a taste of what it would really be like. Plus, you'd be getting paid as well.

"Also, find a mentor in your college program, someone you trust who can advise you. And listen to what they have to say. As they get to know you, they'll get a sense of where you would fit in the best."

●　●　●

FOR MORE INFORMATION

For general information about counseling, as well as information on specialties such as school, college, and career counseling, contact:

> American Counseling Association
> 5999 Stevenson Avenue
> Alexandria, VA 22304

For general information about school counselors, contact:

> American School Counselor Association
> 5999 Stevenson Avenue
> Alexandria, VA 22304

State departments of education can supply information on colleges and universities that offer approved guidance and counseling training for state certification and licensure requirements.

State employment service offices have information about job opportunities and entrance requirements for counselors.

CHAPTER 5 Special Education

EDUCATION

B.A./B.S. Required
Postgraduate Preferred
Other

$$$ SALARY/EARNINGS

$20,000 to $45,000

OVERVIEW

Special education teachers, who are found in lower grades and high schools, instruct students with a variety of disabilities, such as visual and hearing impairments, learning disabilities, and physical disabilities. They work with students from toddlers to those in their early 20s.

Special education teachers design and modify instruction to meet a student's special needs. Teachers also work with students who have other special instructional needs, such as those who are very bright or gifted or those who have limited English proficiency.

Special education teachers are legally required to participate in the development of an Individualized Education Program (IEP) for each special education student. The IEP sets personalized goals for each student and is tailored to a student's individualized learning style and ability. Teachers review the IEP with parents, school administrators, and often the student's general education teacher. Teachers work closely with parents to inform them of their child's progress and suggest techniques to promote learning at home.

Teachers may use films, slides, overhead projectors, and the latest technology in teaching, such as computers, telecommunication systems, and video discs. Telecommunication technology can bring the real world into the classroom. Through telecommunications, American students can communicate with students in other countries to share personal experiences or research projects of interest to both groups. Computers are used in many classroom activities, from helping students solve math problems to learning English as a second language. Teachers must continually update their skills to use the latest technology in the classroom.

Teachers design their classroom presentations to meet student needs and abilities. They also may work with students individually. Teachers assign lessons, give tests, hear oral presentations, and maintain classroom discipline. Teachers observe and evaluate a student's performance and potential. Teachers increasingly are using new assessment methods, such as examining a portfolio of a student's artwork or writing to measure student achievement. Teachers assess the portfolio at the end of a learning period to judge a student's overall progress. They may then provide additional assistance in areas where a student may need help.

Special education teachers may help students with their transition into special vocational training programs, colleges, or a job. Teachers also participate in education conferences and workshops.

Special education teachers work in a variety of settings. Some have their own classrooms and teach classes comprised entirely of special education students; others work as special education resource teachers and offer individualized help to students in general education classrooms; others teach along with general education teachers in classes composed of both general and special education students.

Including school duties performed outside the classroom, many teachers work more than 40 hours a week. Most teachers work the traditional 10-month school year with a 2-month vacation during the summer. Teachers on the 10-month schedule may teach in summer sessions, take other jobs, travel, or pursue other personal interests. Many enroll in college courses or workshops in order to continue their education. Teachers in districts with a year-round schedule typically work eight weeks, are on vacation for one week, and have a five-week midwinter break.

Most states have tenure laws that prevent teachers from being fired without just cause and due process. Teachers may obtain tenure after they have satisfactorily completed a probationary period of teaching, normally three years. Tenure is not a guarantee of a job, but it does provide some security.

TRAINING

All 50 states and the District of Columbia require public school teachers to be certified. Certification is generally for one or several related subjects. Usually certification is granted by the state board of education or a certification advisory committee.

Teachers may be certified to teach the early childhood grades (usually nursery school through grade 3; the elementary grades (grades 1 through 6 or 8); or a special subject, such as reading or music.

In most states, special education teachers receive a credential to teach kindergarten through grade 12. These teachers train in the specialty that they want, such as teaching children with learning disabilities or behavioral disorders.

Almost all states require applicants for teacher certification to be tested for competency in basic skills such as reading and writing, teaching skills, or subject matter proficiency. Almost all require continuing education for renewal of the teacher's certificate. Some require a master's degree.

Many states have reciprocity agreements that make it easier for teachers certified in one state to become certified in another. Teachers may become board certified by successfully completing the National Board for Professional Teaching Standards certification process. This certification is voluntary, but may result in a higher salary.

About 700 colleges and universities across the United States offer programs in special education, including undergraduate, master's, and doctoral programs. Special education teachers usually undergo longer periods of training than general education teachers. Most bachelor's degree programs are four-year programs that include general and specialized courses in special education. However, an increasing number of institutions require a fifth year or other postbaccalaureate preparation.

Courses include educational psychology, legal issues of special education, child growth and development, and knowledge and skills needed for teaching students with disabilities. Some programs require a specialization, such as teaching students with specific learning disabilities. Others offer generalized special education degrees or study in several specialized areas. The last year of the program is usually spent student teaching in a classroom supervised by a certified teacher.

Many states offer alternative teacher certification programs for people who have college training in the subject they will teach but do not have the education courses required for a regular certificate. Alternative certification programs were originally designed to ease teacher shortages in certain subjects, such as mathematics and science. The programs have expanded to attract other people into teaching, including recent college graduates and midcareer changers. In some programs, individuals begin teaching immediately under provisional certification. After working under the close supervision of experienced educators for one or two years while taking education courses outside school hours, they receive regular certification if they have progressed satisfactorily.

Under other programs, college graduates who do not meet certification requirements take only those courses that they lack, and then become certified. This may take one or two semesters of full-time study.

Aspiring teachers who need certification may also enter programs that grant a master's degree in education, as well as certification. States also issue emergency certificates to individuals who do not meet all requirements for a regular certificate when schools cannot hire enough teachers with regular certificates.

The ability to communicate, inspire trust and confidence, and motivate students, by accepting of differences in others, as well as understand their educational and emotional needs, is essential for special education teachers. They also should be organized, dependable, patient, and creative.

Special education teachers can advance to become supervisors or administrators. They may also earn advanced degrees and become instructors in colleges that prepare other special education teachers.

JOB OUTLOOK

Special education teachers held about 388,000 jobs in 1994 in elementary, middle, and secondary schools. The majority of special education teachers were employed in public schools. The rest worked in separate educational facilities—public or private, residential facilities, or in homebound or hospital environments.

Job openings for all teachers are expected to increase substantially by the end of the decade as the large number of teachers now in their 40s and 50s reach retirement age.

Special education teachers have excellent job prospects, as many school districts report shortages of qualified teachers. Positions in rural areas and inner cities are more plentiful than job openings in suburban or wealthy urban areas.

Also, due to the considerable shortages of teachers in these fields, job opportunities may be better in certain specialties such as the following:

Multiple disabilities

Mental retardation

Visual impairment

Learning disabilities

Preschool special education

Special education teachers who are bilingual or have multicultural experience are also needed to work with an increasingly diverse student population.

Employment of special education teachers is expected to increase much faster than the average for all occupations through the year 2005 due to legislation emphasizing training and employment for individuals with disabilities; technological advances resulting in more survivors of accidents and illnesses; and growing public interest in individuals with special needs.

Qualified persons should have little trouble finding a job, due to increased demand for these workers combined with relatively high turnover among special education teachers.

The number of students requiring special education services has been steadily increasing. This trend is expected to continue due to federal legislation that expanded the age range of special education students to include those ages 3 to 21; medical advances that result in more survivors of accidents and illnesses; the postponement of childbirth by more women, resulting in a greater number of premature births and children born with birth defects; and the increase in the general population.

The growing use of inclusive school settings, where special education students are integrated into general education settings, will also necessitate more reliance on special education teachers. The role of special education teachers is expanding to include acting as a consultant to general education teachers, in addition to teaching special education students in resource rooms, general education classrooms, and separate classrooms made up entirely of special education students.

Many special education teachers switch to general education teaching or change careers altogether, often because of job stress associated with teaching special education, particularly excessive paperwork and inadequate administrative support.

SALARIES

Salaries of special education teachers generally follow the same scale as those for general education teachers. According to the National Education Association, the estimated average salary of all teachers was $36,900 in 1995. The estimated average salary for public secondary was $37,800 a year; public elementary school teachers averaged $36,400. Earnings in private schools generally are lower.

Many public school teachers belong to unions, such as the American Federation of Teachers and the National Education Association, that bargain with school systems over wages, hours, and the terms and conditions of employment.

RELATED FIELDS

Special education teachers work with students with disabilities and special needs. Other occupations that help people with disabilities include school psychologists, social workers, speech pathologists, rehabilitation counselors, adapted physical education teachers, and occupational, physical, creative arts, and recreational therapists.

INTERVIEW

Maureen Wright
Teacher of the Visually Handicapped

Maureen Wright is a VH (visually handicapped) teacher at the Texas School for the Blind and Visually Impaired, a residential campus that has an elementary, junior high, and senior high school. The children she works with range in age from 7 to 12.

What the Job's Really Like

"My job is very different from being in a standard elementary school. We focus on what the students' individual needs are as they relate to their visual impairment. Children come to us to catch up on their braille reading and writing skills and to catch up on the new computer technology that helps blind and visually impaired kids stay in school district and eventually go to college. I teach anything that is going to help them keep up to grade level and then we send them back to their school district.

"The average stay is three to four years, although we have many kids who stay with us throughout their entire school career. They live at our school while they're here. A lot of them come to us around the second grade and, if they get caught up, they usually go back to their regular school district around the fifth grade. Sometimes they come back to us again for a short time in high school when the academics really pick up and they need some further assistance.

"With the children who are on grade level we follow the state curriculum. But most of our kids have fallen behind and aren't on grade level. We do whatever it takes to catch them up to where they need to be. We follow an applied curriculum. That means we go through the state curriculum and pick out the items the students need the most to move on. It takes a lot of time for them to learn braille. It takes a lot longer to learn to read in braille than it does to read in print. So we try to abbreviate what they would get normally in their regular school district.

"I have six children in a class at a time and I work with a teacher's aide. Though it seems like a good ratio, within my class of six children, my kids are functioning on three different reading levels, four different math levels, that sort of thing. So it's not like a group and you say, 'class sit down and open up to page number. . . .' They all have their own books, their own special needs.

"It's very challenging. I like finding ways for the children to fit into regular society. A lot of the children grow up being held so separate from other people. They're the blind ones. And they come to us feeling that way, that they're so different. But at our school they're not. Yes, we realize you're blind, but so is everyone else and we're going to do it anyway.

"We're considered an actual school district and because of that we're expected to follow all the standard policies—the report cards and all the other administrative work. And then because we're special ed, we have another whole set of policies to follow so the politics and the paperwork are what I enjoy the least."

How Maureen Wright Got Started

"I started a little different from most. My grandfather is blind and he taught me to read and write braille when I was only ten years old. I was always driven toward this work; I just sort of grew into the job naturally.

"I have a B.A. in special education with an additional certification in teaching the blind and visually impaired from D'Youville College in Buffalo, New York.

"I started at the Texas School in 1988. I also taught in Manor, Texas, before that at the State School. Back in the mid-'80s handicapped children were in the state hospital schools and then the law required Texas to get the children out of the state hospitals into the regular school districts. My job was to teach them to be socially appropriate enough so they'd be able to function in the regular schools."

Expert Advice

"My suggestion would be to go and volunteer at one of the schools before you begin your studies. I don't think most people realize what's involved. We get student teachers who come work with us for three or four weeks. It's their first experience at the school and then they realize that, boy, this isn't what they want to do at all. Schools like ours all over the country are begging for volunteers. It would only take one phone call to set something up.

"And of course, the obvious, you have to love kids. But one thing I've noticed is that many people come in to volunteer who are so tenderhearted, so sweet. They have so many feelings for these poor, blind children. But they don't realize that the kind of people we need in this work are those who can look at the children and see them as just any other kids. If they do something wrong, you have to tell them 'no, it's wrong.' Just because they're blind, they can't get away with things.

"And helping them too much in some cases is the worst possible thing you could do. You need to let them find their own way, you need to let them fall or fail or bump into walls once in a while. This is all under very careful supervision, of course, but the children need to understand that hands don't come out of midair to save them all the time. You need to be tough enough to let the children learn on their own sometimes."

● ● ●

INTERVIEW

Janice M. Lee
Specialist for the Learning Disabled (Graduate Intern)

Janice M. Lee is a graduate intern at SUNY–Binghamton's Services for Students with Disabilities. In 1994 she earned her B.A. in Literature and Language and in 1996 her Master of Arts in Social Sciences, both from State University of New York at Binghamton.

What the Job's Really Like

"I have so many titles and responsibilities it's hard to pin them down. Primarily I'm an instructor. I teach college students who have attention deficit disorder, learning disabilities, and head injuries both in one-on-one tutorial sessions and in small class settings.

"Secondly I'm their coach, counselor, and confidante. Many come in and cry on my shoulder when the going gets rough. I calm them down, listen to their pain, then point out their strengths and how they've pulled them through tough spots before. By that time the student is thinking more positively and we brainstorm how to survive this crisis.

"I also review student documentation, since my supervisor is primarily versed in medical and mobility impairments. I've had a lot of the tests I go over due to a head injury I sustained four years ago, so I have far more than a working knowledge of what they're about. I remember what they looked like and how tedious they were to take.

"On top of all of this I supervise the undergraduate intern who acts as our Adaptive Computer Lab Manager. With my computer background, I'm more likely to know what is happening in the lab and what needs to be done. Plus, I research administrative software, order it, then teach our secretary and supervisor how to use it once it has been installed. And I've had to become proficient in using the adaptive computer software so I can help train incoming lab managers and students. I've learned to use a voice-activated program called Kurzweil and another program for our dyslexics called Word Scholar that has great look-up functions. If you can't remember a whole word, no problem. Put in what you know and it comes back with all the possibilities. Spell words inside out or phonetically? No problem. Type it in the way you normally do, and the program runs all the possible permutations of those letters till you pick out the word you wanted. It's time consuming to learn these programs, but well worth it. Using them can make an enormous difference in a student's ability to succeed in the world of academia.

"There is no such thing as a typical day. Yes, certain things remain the same, such as the times I hold classes or have my own classes and the times for staff meetings. I try to schedule students for tutoring or coaching at regular times so they remember and so no one ever gets scheduled in the wrong time slot. After that my world at the office is up in the air.

"A typical day might go something like this: I come in around 9:00 A.M. I hate mornings and early rising, but such is life. . . . Usually, I have a whole of two seconds to myself before

Jean Fairbairn, my supervisor, is calling me into her office. She just got a student's documentation or something she has to deal with that day and wants a second take on it. I grab it and walk it to my desk, picking up the messages and info crammed into my folder on the filing cabinet. I sit down, arrange my belongings, and review the 'urgent' material.

"If it's a day that I teach, I try to spend half an hour before class going over my lesson plan and making sure I have all copies of handouts made and in folders to go.

"Inevitably a student pops his or her head in the door at the last minute to say hi. If he or she is in my class, we walk upstairs together. We chat. With all the roles I have to juggle, I decided that my primary role must be friend. It blankets all the rest in a wonderfully inclusive way.

"I teach for an hour, usually doing far more facilitating than lecturing. I believe strongly in collaborative learning, especially with my students. They learn far more from one another than I could ever hope to teach them. I just provide them with the topic, resources, and motivation. The biggest thing they learn in my classes is that they aren't alone, they aren't stupid and that there are things they can do to make their learning easier. They also learn that I don't take myself seriously. I will joke around, and if you go over my limit you may find a chalk eraser flying in your general direction.

"Once class is over I generally have a tutoring or coaching session afterwards. These students need constant feedback on their struggles and achievements. They feel so all alone with their problems. They need to know that there's an instructor out there who understands their frustrations and has the patience to go the distance with them. I try my darndest to be that instructor.

"I force myself to take time out for lunch. The first two semesters I would allow people to so control my day that I often found myself forgetting to eat. A lot of times I'll go to lunch with one of the students who uses our office (not necessarily a student from my class). This gets me out of the office and gives me a little breather.

"One day a week the entire staff has a meeting. I hate them. I'm not an administrator. But I dig in because I know that my supervisor really needs to keep a handle on everything that's going on and she needs our input.

"One day a week Jean and I have a one-on-one meeting over lunch. We ramble and get on all sorts of subjects. Sometimes we get stuck on one student who is having real struggles and try to decide how we can best help him or her and what resources are available on campus. I enjoy these meetings. Jean is the best supervisor I've ever had. To her everyone is absolutely necessary and she'd about die if she lost any of the workers in her office. She really treasures her people and we all feel it and work for her in a way we wouldn't in some other office. I've never had so much appreciation from a supervisor before in all my life.

"It's hard to get out of the office. Jean is capable of stopping my outward rush with an urgent phone call I just have to take or a briefing for a meeting the next day. But I try hard to keep my schedule solid. This kind of work can burn you out fast if you don't take some time out for yourself.

"Our office is 100 percent cooperative. No one works against anyone else. I really love my students. You have to spend time with them to understand just how great it is, but when you have a student come up and tell you they don't know how they would have gotten through the semester without you, a glow builds up inside and you know that all of your efforts meant something. I really feel like I'm making a difference in people's lives. I can see people grow as I work with them and that brings a high better than any drug.

"The LD and ADD students are some of the hardest-working people you'll ever meet in your life. They work and struggle and persist until they finally understand the material and have a quality product to show for it. Sometimes their efforts are nothing short of heroic. I have immense respect and admiration for them. Plus, they're very appreciative of everything someone does to help them. I bond strongly with them and they with me. You don't get the same quality of students and relationships between instructor and student that you get with students with LDs and ADD."

How Janice M. Lee Got Started

"I earned my B.A. in Literature and Language and fully expected to go into English and become a professor. But that profession is closing down and there are as many as 1,000 applicants for every professorial position. I knew I had to shift gears in order to make my degree meaningful.

"I had used the disabilities office on campus because of neurological problems due to a head injury I'd received a couple of years before. The director kept telling me about this graduate internship they were going to have open in the fall and that she was looking for someone with a strong English background. It was a plus that I also had a degree and experience with computers and knowledge of learning disabilities.

"I have a daughter who has attention deficit disorder and a hearing perception problem. I've learned from my experience with her and the training I've gotten from her psychologists.

"For the past two years I have been involved in a unique master's program that essentially allows me to create my own degree within the social sciences arena and within certain boundaries and guidelines set down by the Human Development Department at SUNY–Binghamton. For the 1994–1995 school year I continued with graduate English courses, particularly Teaching of College English and Teaching of College Writing. During the 1995–1996 school year I concentrated more heavily on counseling skills, taking an overview of the history and schools of counseling theory and a course this spring in which we got specific instruction and practice in small groups in counseling.

"Last fall I also took an independent study that I felt was necessary to understand learning disabilities and ADD: Neuropsychology and the Diagnosis of Learning Disorders. This spring I took a second independent study course in which I wrote a reference manual for all of the psycho-educational documentation that students must present to document their disabilities.

"This fall, for my integrative seminar (similar to a master's thesis), I will be designing a learning center for college students with disabilities.

"Nothing can prepare you for a job better than hands-on experience, and I've been getting more than my share of that for the past two years and loving every minute of it."

Expert Advice

"First and foremost, to work with these students you have to be a strong person. Your own self-esteem has to be very, very high because you must be genuine, sincere, and vulnerable. These students pick up on phoniness faster than a bloodhound on a trail. They turn against you if they think you're just patronizing them.

"Really search your heart to find the person you are first. You must know that you want to help these students even if it means sacrificing time, energy, and personal resources. Can you really do that? If you can, then consider the next criterion. You need more patience for these guys than for any toddler. A toddler you expect to be rambunctious, full of energy, and inconsistent. When you have a 20- or 30-year old sitting across from you who acts more like a toddler at times, the incongruity can be a real jolt to your psyche. One day they're following their academic plan, the next day they've completely screwed it up. One day they're high because something finally came together and made sense for them. The next day they're resistant to even trying something new that could make a world of difference to their ability to learn.

"If you can juggle mentally and emotionally and stay on an even keel, then go for it!"

● ● ●

INTERVIEW

Lynne Robbins
Elementary Special Education Teacher

Lynne Robbins is a special education teacher at the William Monroe Trotter School, an elementary school in Boston, Massachusetts. She studied at Bennington College in Vermont and earned her B.A. in psychology with a concentration in art. She earned her M.Ed. at Boston College in special education and most recently her Master of Science in Art Education (M.S.A.E.) from Massachusetts College of Art in 1996.

What the Job's Really Like

"I work with special education children in grades 1 through 5 as well as with regular education children in integrated classrooms.

"I am a certified art teacher, special education teacher, and elementary teacher. I have taught in several fields beginning with multiple handicapped deaf children through to adolescents with multiple handicaps and deafness. I then switched to working with disadvantaged children in the inner city schools.

"I have a background as an artist (mixed media, metals, textbook illustration, advertising) and most of what I do as a teacher involves the same processes. Teaching is a very creative profession. It involves working with ideas and making them take root in reality. For example, a recent project with students involved studying solar energy and then creating solar cars and solar-powered vehicles, painting and decorating them. The project grew into an immense undertaking that involved eight adults and over 125 children, and which may become an after-school institute.

"Artmaking is a problem-solving process; so is science. I believe that similarities go beyond differences conceptually. We have made artist's books, learned to write through art, created murals, used multimedia. The list is endless. Most students love to work in this manner—and the enthusiasm is often quite high.

"A typical day involves working with 22 learning handicapped children during six or seven block periods. Most are 'pulled out' from their regular classes; sometimes I work with them in the classroom, along with the entire class.

"The pace is frantic, the day flies by. It's never boring, sometimes relaxing, though usually totally unpredictable. There's always something new to do or to learn with the students.

"The city of Boston, as well as the country, is working with new goals, standards for education. There is a lot of curriculum change, innovation—all the elements that artists love—challenge, innovation, problems to solve, materials to utilize. I call my work creating with a human canvas.

"Currently some students are creating books by using throwaway cameras, getting prints, creating chapter heads, writing 'pitchlines' of 15 words or less for chapters, editing them for spelling (using process writing procedures), and then we have them bound into hardcover books. Some students may be doing independent research projects using the Internet on computers that were purchased through arts-based grants.

"Others may be using multimedia arts programs (Flying Colors, Amazing Writing Machine) to create individual books/art work/projects. Most of the work is monitored by goals and objectives for 766 (the special ed law), individualized for each student. Most projects take between three to six weeks.

"The teaching day goes from 9:00 A.M. to 3:30 P.M. I often use time after school to coach students or to do an after-school class or projects in the district. There are always workshops available for teachers, lots of opportunities for professional growth and development.

"My job is infinitely creative. It is challenging, process-oriented, unpredictable due to human factors; one never knows what the next minute or hour might bring.

"The projects, which are arts or science based, are creative in scope and thus fascinating for me to develop and to implement. I often need to get grants, write them, have them funded. My school is multicultural, primarily Black and Asian—and I enjoy the challenge and pleasures of working with people of various cultural backgrounds.

"My current hang-up about my work is that there is never enough time to do all we want to. The work is demanding, exhausting, and sometimes I wish there were a little less stress associated with it.

"But working with children and their parents has brought me a great deal of personal happiness and joy. I can see myself working as an educator forever."

How Lynne Robbins Got Started

"I am an artist. I visited the classroom of a gifted teacher at a Headstart program in Vermont when I was at Bennington. There was no money but they were rich in ideas; brushes were made from sponges and branches and blocks from lumber scraps and pegs. The children were happy, busy. I thought the teacher a miracle worker. I wanted to be one, too.

"I switched my major from art to psychology with a concentration in art. I didn't know precisely what direction to go in. When I took my first job it was possible for employees to apply for graduate school there at lower rates. I took advantage of this to take the GREs, passed them, and enrolled in the grad program.

"I kind of stumbled into special education, then into art as an art teacher with various programs (museum or community-based or summer schools), and finally began using art no matter where I was stationed or in what capacity because it was a part of me, and the way I functioned best.

"I also stumbled into my first job through a summer camp job as an art teacher at a behavior mod camp and a chance encounter with a social worker. It was at a campus lab school for handicapped children. I worked as a teacher's assistant for a regular class and as an art teacher for the entire school. I'll never forget the day some of the wheelchair kids deliberately tipped over cans of paint and wheeled through them, streaking the corridors with all manner of color tracks. It didn't hurt that they also grabbed brushes and streaked the walls as they went. I thought I would die on the spot.

"I worked with deaf and multiple handicapped children and adults for nine years. The secret of my teaching was my base as an artist. I held jobs in both Massachusetts and California, working with private schools, private programs, community colleges.

"Then, I burned out and took off about four years to work as a freelancer and ad artist. At the same time, I went back to school to receive certification in art education so that I could work as an art teacher in the public schools. My training and student teaching were exciting; my elementary classes gave me a standing ovation and my high school classes were exhilarating.

"When I learned Boston was looking for teachers, I applied as a special education teacher to get into the system. My assignments were as an elementary moderate special needs teacher. However, my art training was not in vain—most of my projects with students were arts based and received recognition both for the students and myself.

"I am now contemplating working as an art teacher, since there are several new pilot projects in the city that look very appealing."

Expert Advice

"If you want to teach, you will need to reach down deep inside yourself and ask yourself if you have the stamina, the commitment, the creativity, and the endurance.

"The challenge for me has come from the fact that I happen to be deaf, and am working with hearing students, which has made for many a hairy and hair-raising experience. It has been a personal journey for me, as well as a professional one—learning to deal with the nature of the beast.

"Teaching has been a struggle for me, because it exposed me to the best and worse of human nature on a daily basis—my own and others! It will call for everything you have. It will demand that you draw on resources that you didn't know existed, mental, spiritual, emotional. The payoff will come from knowing that you can make a difference in the lives of many individuals.

"I found it's also important to have structure of sorts, to be able to structure even the most creative of projects, at least externally—because special ed students often work best from a structured base, going from structure to creativity.

"Special education students are not necessarily the Brady Bunch—you'll need a great deal of patience and tolerance, and a sense of humor."

●   ●   ●

INTERVIEW

Elyse Feldman
Educational Therapist

Elyse Feldman earned her B.A. in education from Hunter College (New York City) in 1967 with a teaching license in fine arts. Her master's was in special education in 1972, also from Hunter. She works part time with an organization called Women in Need and also has a private practice working with people with learning disabilities. She has been in this profession since the early 1970s.

What the Job's Really Like

"Women in Need is an organization for women who have hit bottom. They are just coming out of years of substance abuse. They have lost their children to foster care and most are living in shelters. WIN's program runs about a year and a half, and in that time the women receive therapy, parenting classes, health education, and academic education. Most of them have not graduated from high school. I am the only educational therapist at this site but I have volunteers who work with me.

"My job title at WIN varies with the wind. I'm listed in the books as an Educational Consultant and Independent Contractor. I do whatever comes up. I teach GED topics and provide vocational counseling. Each student gets her own particular agenda based on her needs—as far as I can furnish them."

"I am there two days a week. I work with clients on an individual basis since every one is on a different level. Most of the students are very afraid of the classroom situation because of various bad experiences—so I am mother, bully, cajoler, God, ear, magician, hugger, huggee—you name it.

"The class size can go from 1 to 18. Not all finish the program. I lose a lot of them along the way. They relapse. Some have died from AIDS, many are HIV positive, some only stay until housing is found for them, and so on.

"I've learned to take each day as it comes. I've taught so long now that my 'bag of tricks' is full and I can cope with most situations that come up. I work there about 14 hours a week. I'm never bored. There's always some calamity afoot.

"The unfortunate part of my working there is that as a part-time worker, nobody gives you citizenship, so to speak. They forget to tell you things you should know—most of the other staff are overworked and underpaid. Often I'm the last to know many things and it has made for a great deal of frustration. Communication gaps are huge. Many of the staff have come and gone in the time I've been there, and because WIN is an organization dependent upon the kindness of strangers with money, it is at the mercy of people who don't know anything about our clients. They just send directives.

"They're wonderful, funny, brave, and loving, and they've taught me a lot. I've seen miracles happen in my room.

"I also have a private practice. It started with youngsters, back in the '80s, then a woman in her forties was referred to me. She was a classic dyslexic and I was intrigued and started to research intensely in this area and my practice took on a whole new slant. I also found that working with adults was more interesting to me. Now much of what I do is counseling, trying to separate the "disease" from the defensive behaviors surrounding it.

"I am getting more and more clients who are realizing that they are learning disabled by virtue of their having attention deficit disorder. Here, memory, or the lack of it, is a great factor—and a huge problem to overcome—especially so with clients whose brains have been a bit fried from drug or alcohol abuse.

"What is often required is learning a whole gestalt of the clients' life attitudes—and then starting to slowly help them focus on one thing at a time, to prioritize what is most important to them, and then to set up a series or an outline of actions. It is goal-oriented, mentor- or coach-oriented work."

How Elyse Feldman Got Started

"Altruism did not enter the picture. Rather it was a misguided notion that teaching, my original goal, was a 'safe' and solid kind of career to have. When I started college (CCNY) I was a drama major but I left it, and school, when I found out how much undressing of one's soul was involved. And I didn't have the ego for it. Ergo, I became an English major at Lehman College in the Bronx. The teachers I encountered there were so unbelievably awful and unsupportive that I left there and didn't go back to college for another few years.

"My next try was at Hunter, where I had decided that teaching art sounded like a 'safe' and solid move. Little did I know I'd be asked to be mother, doctor, God, ear, comforter, policewoman (taking knives away from students). Things had changed a bit since I had gone to junior high school.

"I got my first job in the junior high school I had attended. When I went for my interview, carrying my art portfolio, I was informed that the position was filled. As I was leaving the art department, the head said, 'Why don't you see Mrs. B in the English department. They need a teacher there.' Mrs. B interviewed me. I told her my license was in art. She said, 'What do you think could be your qualifications for teaching English?' I said, 'I speak it.' I was hired.

"In 1969 I began to teach in a very special school called The Livingston School for Girls. They were girls who had been thrown out of every other school in the city and they were really rough. I think I stayed scared for the full first year I was there.

But the principal was a genius (the author of a book about the school, *The Angel Inside Went Sour*), and I learned a great deal.

"From 1971 to 1975 the principal received a grant to start the first New York City Crisis Hotline for our students, which then grew to include parents, friends, and strangers. The next grant we received was to run a Hot Line for teachers, the only one I've ever heard about, and much needed. I ran workshops, taught teachers how to handle difficult school situations, manned the phones, and held private sessions with teachers in crisis."

Expert Advice

"Teaching is not about giving answers and it's not about how much information you have to offer them. It's about opening doors, holding hands, being patient, not having your own private agenda for your students, not being disappointed or hurt when they don't reach your expectations and hopes. Leave your ego at the door. Learn to ask wonderful questions that allow them to think. Make sure they know that one of the most productive things they can do is 'fail.' Some students are so paralyzed by the idea of failure that they won't even try. Applaud every strength you find in them. Go with what they know. Address them by name. Know that sarcasm doesn't work and respect will.

"If you find that there's a student you just can't stand, look inside yourself. I think you will find that you are angry at the student because he or she is not doing what you want him or her to do. If it's important for you to be in control and your natural style is an authoritarian one, teach college instead.

"With counseling, try not to label and box your clients into a category; it will stop you from thinking creatively. Make sure both you and the client agree on what is needed and wanted. A holistic approach for the client's mental and physical health is best.

"Symptoms here can be very tricky and sometimes it's very difficult to tell if it's hormonal, nutritional, psychological, or genetic. Therefore, a good physical, psychological, and educational workup is in order before you start working with the client. Also, because this type of client most often has a background of isolation and hiding, it is helpful if they can get involved in doing group work with others who are dealing with the same or similar difficulties."

● ● ●

FOR MORE INFORMATION

For information on a career as a special education teacher, a list of accredited institutions offering training programs in special education and financial aid information may be obtained from:

> National Clearinghouse for Professions in Special Education
> Council for Exceptional Children
> 1920 Association Drive
> Reston, VA 22091

Information on certification requirements and approved teacher training institutions is available from local school systems and state departments of education.

Information on teachers' unions and education-related issues may be obtained from:

> American Federation of Teachers
> 555 New Jersey Avenue NW
> Washington, DC 20001

> National Education Association
> 1201 16th Street NW
> Washington, DC 20036

A list of institutions with teacher education programs accredited by the National Council for Accreditation of Teacher Education can be obtained from:

> National Council for Accreditation of Teacher Education
> 2010 Massachusetts Avenue NW, 2nd Floor
> Washington, DC 20036

For information on voluntary teacher certification requirements, contact:

> National Board for Professional Teaching Standards
> 300 River Place
> Detroit, MI 48207

CHAPTER 6 Psychologists

EDUCATION
Postgraduate Required

$$$ SALARY/EARNINGS
$26,000 to $100,000

OVERVIEW

Psychologists study human behavior and mental processes to understand, explain, and change people's behavior. They may study the way a person thinks, feels, or behaves. Research psychologists investigate the physical, cognitive, emotional, or social aspects of human behavior. Like other social scientists, psychologists formulate hypotheses and collect data to test their validity. Research methods depend on the topic under study. Psychologists may gather information through controlled laboratory experiments; personality, performance, aptitude, and intelligence tests; observation, interviews, and questionnaires; clinical studies; or surveys. Computers are widely used to record and analyze this information.

Psychologists in applied fields counsel and conduct training programs; do market research; apply psychological treatments to a variety of medical and surgical conditions; or provide mental health services in hospitals, clinics, or private settings.

Because psychology deals with human behavior, psychologists apply their knowledge and techniques to a wide range of endeavors including human services, management, education, law, and sports.

In addition to the variety of work settings, psychologists specialize in many different areas.

CLINICAL PSYCHOLOGISTS, who constitute the largest specialty, generally work in independent or group practice or in hospitals or clinics. They may help the mentally or emotionally disturbed adjust to life and are increasingly helping all kinds of medical and surgical patients deal with their illnesses or injuries. They may work in physical medicine and rehabilitation settings, treating patients with spinal cord injuries, chronic pain or illness, stroke, and arthritis and neurologic conditions, such as multiple sclerosis. Others help people deal with life stresses such as divorce or aging.

Clinical Psychologists interview patients; give diagnostic tests; provide individual, family, and group psychotherapy; and design and implement behavior modification programs. They may collaborate with physicians and other specialists in developing treatment programs and help patients understand and comply with the prescribed treatment.

Some clinical psychologists work in universities, where they train graduate students in the delivery of mental health and behavioral medicine services. Others administer community mental health programs.

COUNSELING PSYCHOLOGISTS perform many of the same functions as clinical psychologists, and use several techniques, including interviewing and testing, to advise people on how to deal with problems of everyday living—personal, social, educational, or vocational.

DEVELOPMENTAL PSYCHOLOGISTS study the patterns and causes of behavioral change as people progress through life from infancy to adulthood. Some concern themselves with behavior during infancy, childhood, and adolescence, while others study changes that take place during maturity and old age. The study of developmental disabilities and how they affect a person and others is a new area within developmental psychology.

EDUCATIONAL PSYCHOLOGISTS evaluate student and teacher needs, and design and develop programs to enhance the educational setting.

EXPERIMENTAL PSYCHOLOGISTS study behavior processes and work with human beings and animals such as rats, monkeys, and pigeons. Prominent areas of experimental research include motivation, thinking, attention, learning and retention, sensory and perceptual processes, effects of substance use and abuse, and genetic and neurological factors in behavior.

INDUSTRIAL AND ORGANIZATIONAL PSYCHOLOGISTS apply psychological techniques to personnel administration, management, and marketing problems. They are involved in policy planning, applicant screening, training and development, psychological test research, counseling, and organizational development and analysis. For example, an industrial psychologist may work with management to develop better training programs and to reorganize the work setting to improve worker productivity or quality of worklife.

SCHOOL PSYCHOLOGISTS work with students, teachers, parents, and administrators to resolve students' learning and behavior problems. Social psychologists examine people's interactions with others and with the social environment. Prominent areas of study include group behavior, leadership, attitudes, and interpersonal perception.

Some relatively new specialties include the following:

COGNITIVE PSYCHOLOGISTS deal with the brain's role in memory, thinking, and perceptions; some are involved with research related to computer programming and artificial intelligence.

HEALTH PSYCHOLOGISTS promote good health through health maintenance counseling programs that are designed, for example, to help people stop smoking or lose weight.

NEUROPSYCHOLOGISTS study the relationship between the brain and behavior. They often work in stroke and head injury programs.

GEROPSYCHOLOGISTS deal with the special problems faced by the elderly. The emergence and growth of these specialties reflects the increasing participation of psychologists in providing direct services to special patient populations.

Other areas of specialization include psychometrics, psychology and the arts, history of psychology, psychopharmacology, community, comparative, consumer, engineering, environmental, family, forensic, population, military, and rehabilitation psychology.

Besides the jobs described above, many persons hold positions as psychology faculty at colleges and universities, and as high school psychology teachers.

A psychologist's specialty and place of employment determine working conditions. For example, clinical, school, and counseling psychologists in private practice have pleasant, comfortable offices and set their own hours. However, they often have evening hours to accommodate their clients.

Some employed in hospitals, nursing homes, and other health facilities often work evenings and weekends, while others in schools and clinics work regular hours.

Psychologists employed by academic institutions divide their time among teaching, research, and administrative responsibilities. Some maintain part-time consulting practices as well.

In contrast to the many psychologists who have flexible work schedules, most in government and private industry have more structured schedules. Reading and writing research reports, they often work alone. Many experience the pressures of deadlines, tight schedules, and overtime work. Their routines may be interrupted frequently. Travel may be required to attend conferences or conduct research.

After several years of experience, some psychologists—usually those with doctoral degrees—enter private practice or set up their own research or consulting firms. A growing proportion of psychologists are self-employed.

TRAINING

A doctoral degree generally is required for employment as a psychologist. Psychologists with a Ph.D. qualify for a wide range of teaching, research, clinical, and counseling positions in universities, elementary and secondary schools, private industry, and government.

Psychologists with a Psy.D. (Doctor of Psychology) qualify mainly for clinical positions.

Persons with a master's degree in psychology can administer tests as psychological assistants. Under the supervision of doctoral level psychologists, they can conduct research in laboratories, conduct psychological evaluations, counsel patients, or perform administrative duties. They may teach in high schools or two-year colleges or work as school psychologists or counselors.

A bachelor's degree in psychology qualifies a person to assist psychologists and other professionals in community mental health centers, vocational rehabilitation offices, and correctional programs; to work as research or administrative assistants; and to take jobs as trainees in government or business. However, without additional academic training, their advancement opportunities in psychology are severely limited.

In the federal government, candidates having at least 24 semester hours in psychology and one course in statistics qualify for entry-level positions. Competition for these jobs is keen, however. Clinical psychologists generally must have completed the Ph.D. or Psy.D. requirements and have served an internship; vocational and guidance counselors usually need two years of graduate study in counseling and one year of counseling experience.

In most cases, two years of full-time graduate study are needed to earn a master's degree in psychology. Requirements usually include practical experience in an applied setting or a master's thesis based on a research project. A master's degree in school psychology requires about two years of course work and a one-year internship.

Five to seven years of graduate work usually are required for a doctoral degree. The Ph.D. degree culminates in a dissertation based on original research. Courses in quantitative research methods, which include the use of computers, are an integral part of graduate study and usually necessary to complete the dissertation.

The Psy.D. usually is based on practical work and examinations rather than a dissertation. In clinical or counseling psychology, the requirements for the doctoral degree generally include a year or more of internship or supervised experience.

Competition for admission into most graduate programs is keen. Some universities require an undergraduate major in psychology. Others prefer only basic psychology with courses in the biological, physical, and social sciences, statistics, and mathematics.

Most colleges and universities offer a bachelor's degree program in psychology; several hundred offer a master's and/or a Ph.D. program. A relatively small number of professional schools of psychology—some affiliated with colleges or universities, offer the Psy.D.

The American Psychological Association (APA) presently accredits doctoral training programs in clinical, counseling, and school psychology. The National Council for Accreditation of Teacher Education, with the assistance of the National Association of School Psychologists, also is involved in the accreditation of advanced degree programs in school psychology. APA also accredits institutions that provide internships for doctoral students in school, clinical, and counseling psychology.

Although financial aid is difficult to obtain, some universities award fellowships or scholarships or arrange for part-time employment. The Veterans Administration (VA) offers predoctoral traineeships to interns in VA hospitals, clinics, and related training agencies. The National Science Foundation, the Department of Health and Human Services, and many other organizations also provide grants to psychology departments to help fund student stipends.

Psychologists in independent practice or those who offer any type of patient care, including clinical, counseling, and school psychologists, must meet certification or licensing requirements. All states and the District of Columbia have such requirements.

Licensing laws vary by state, but generally require a doctorate in psychology, completion of an approved internship, and one to two years of professional experience. In addition, most states require that applicants pass an examination. Most state boards administer a standardized test and, in many instances, additional oral or essay examinations. Very few states certify those with a master's degree as psychological assistants or associates. Some states require continuing education for license renewal.

Most states require that licensed or certified psychologists limit their practice to those areas in which they have developed professional competence through training and experience.

The American Board of Professional Psychology recognizes professional achievement by awarding diplomas—primarily in clinical psychology, clinical neuropsychology, counseling, forensic, industrial and organizational, and school psychology. Candidates need a doctorate in psychology, five years of experience, and professional endorsements; they also must pass an examination.

Even more than in other occupations, aspiring psychologists who are interested in direct patient care must be emotionally stable, mature, and able to deal effectively with people. Sensitivity, compassion, and the ability to lead and inspire others are particularly important for clinical work and counseling. Research psychologists should be able to do detailed work independently and as part of a team. Verbal and writing skills are necessary to communicate treatment and research findings. Patience and perseverance are vital qualities because results from psychological treatment of patients or research often are long in coming.

JOB OUTLOOK

Psychologists held about 144,000 jobs in 1994. Educational institutions employed nearly 4 out of 10 salaried psychologists in positions involving counseling, testing, special education, research, and administration; hospitals, mental health clinics, rehabilitation centers, nursing homes, and other health facilities employed 3 out of 10; and government agencies at the federal, state, and local levels employed one-sixth. The Department of Veterans Affairs, the Department of Defense, and the Public Health Service employ the overwhelming majority of psychologists working for federal agencies. Governments employ psychologists in hospitals, clinics, correctional facilities, and other settings. Psychologists also work in social service organizations, research organizations, management consulting firms, marketing research firms, and other businesses.

Employment of psychologists is expected to grow faster than the average for all occupations through the year 2005. Largely because of the substantial investment in training required to enter this specialized field, psychologists have a strong attachment to their occupation—only a relatively small proportion leave the profession each year. Nevertheless, replacement needs are expected to account for most job openings, similar to most occupations.

Programs to combat the increases in alcohol abuse, drug dependency, marital strife, family violence, crime, and other problems plaguing society should stimulate employment growth. Other factors spurring demand for psychologists include increased emphasis on mental health maintenance in conjunction with the treatment of physical illness; public concern for the development of human resources, including the growing elderly population; increased testing and counseling of children; and more interest in rehabilitation of prisoners. Changes in the level of government funding for these kinds of services could affect the demand for psychologists.

Job opportunities in health care should remain strong, particularly in health care provider networks, such as health maintenance and preferred provider organizations, that specialize in mental health, and in nursing homes and alcohol and drug abuse rehabilitation programs. Job opportunities will arise in businesses, nonprofit organizations, and research and computer firms. Companies will use psychologists' expertise in survey design, analysis, and research to provide personnel testing, program evaluation, and statistical analysis. The increase in employee assistance programs in which psychologists help people stop smoking, control weight, or alter other behaviors also should spur job growth. The expected wave of retirements among college faculty, beginning in the late 1990s, should result in job openings for psychologists in colleges and universities.

Other openings are likely to occur as psychologists study the effectiveness of changes in health, education, military, law enforcement, and consumer protection programs. Psychologists also are increasingly studying the effects on people of technological advances in areas such as agriculture, energy, the conservation and use of natural resources, and industrial and office automation.

Opportunities are best for candidates with a doctoral degree. Persons holding doctorates from leading universities in applied areas such as school, clinical, counseling, health, industrial, and educational psychology should have particularly good prospects.

Psychologists with extensive training in quantitative research methods and computer science may have a competitive edge over applicants without this background.

Graduates with a master's degree in psychology may encounter competition for the limited number of jobs for which they qualify.

Graduates of master's degree programs in school psychology should have the best job prospects, as schools are expected to increase student counseling and mental health services. Some master's degree holders may find jobs as psychological assistants in community mental health centers. These positions often require direct supervision by a licensed psychologist. (See Chapter 3.)

Others may find jobs involving research and data collection and analysis in universities, government, or private companies.

Bachelor's degree holders can expect very few opportunities directly related to psychology. Some may find jobs as assistants in rehabilitation centers or in other jobs involving data collection and analysis.

Those who meet state certification requirements may become high school psychology teachers.

SALARIES

According to a 1993 survey by the American Psychological Association, the median annual salary of psychologists with a doctoral degree was $39,100 in counseling psychology; $39,000 in research positions; $40,000 in clinical psychology; and $45,000 in school psychology. In an earlier survey median annual salaries in industrial/organizational psychology were $76,000; in university psychology departments, median annual salaries ranged from $32,000 for assistant professors to $55,000 for full professors.

The median annual salary of master's degree holders was $35,000 for faculty; $26,000 in counseling psychology; $24,000 in clinical psychology; $28,000 in research positions; $58,000 in industrial/organizational psychology; and $34,500 in school psychology. Some psychologists have much higher earnings, particularly those in private practice.

The federal government recognizes education and experience in certifying applicants for entry-level positions. In general, the average starting salary for psychologists having a bachelor's degree was about $18,700 a year in 1995; those with superior academic records could begin at $23,200. Counseling and school psychologists with a master's degree and one year of counseling experience could start at $28,300. Clinical psychologists having a Ph.D. or Psy.D. degree and one year of internship could start at $34,300; some individuals could start at $41,100.

The average salary for psychologists in the federal government in nonsupervisory, supervisory, and managerial positions was about $58,300 a year in 1995.

RELATED FIELDS

Psychologists are trained to conduct research and teach, evaluate, counsel, and advise individuals and groups with special needs. Others who do this kind of work include psychiatrists, social workers, sociologists, clergy, special education teachers, and counselors.

INTERVIEW

Gerald D. Oster
Clinical Psychologist

Gerald D. Oster is a licensed psychologist with a private practice. He is also a clinical associate professor of psychiatry at the University of Maryland Medical School in Baltimore.

He earned his B.A. in sociology at the University of South Florida, Tampa in 1971; his M.A. in psychology at Middle Tennessee State University in Murfreesboro in 1976; and his Ph.D. in psychology at Virginia Commonwealth University in Richmond in 1981.

What the Job's Really Like

"Since I have decided to have several jobs—and this was a conscious decision because I'm primarily a person who enjoys variety—my days also vary. For instance, Tuesday mornings find me for two hours at a community mental health center in the inner city of Baltimore, where I work as a child and family therapist. Right now I'm working with two particular patients. One is a 16-year-old youth who had trouble with the law. He served time in juvenile delinquent centers and now is trying to make it back into the community but is struggling to fit in at school and in his foster care placement.

"The other is a child in kindergarten who is very insecure about the world about him. He lives in a very dangerous neighborhood with his grandparents as his primary caretakers. His mother, who also lives with him, is a drug addict.

"When I am not seeing these two patients, I am doing the enormous paperwork required by the various governing agencies that monitor the clinic.

"After catching up at the clinic (I work at home and in my private practice on Mondays), I spend an eight-hour period at the University Counseling Center, where I see the opposite of the spectrum—very intelligent and creative individuals who are in various professional schools (law, medicine, social work, etc.). Although quite articulate and resourceful, they, too, have their own struggles and often make good use of the support that our Center provides. Usually, they come to us due to the stress of school, but also due to life's complications, meaning problems in relationships, caretaking of others (many are married or have relatives or children that they are responsible for). Also, the pace and expectations for learning are incredible and require a huge sacrifice socially that many have a difficult time adjusting to. After these hours are over, I usually go to my private practice to sort through the mail or see an occasional evening patient.

"My other days are similar but involve different demands and different populations each day. Sometimes I am at the local community hospital interviewing or testing a suicidal or out-of-control adolescent. My private practice is divided between seeing children and adults with an assortment of problems that might stem from family discord, learning difficulties in school and their emotional impact, and relationship problems (of which there are many variations).

"I stay quite busy, but always have to seek out new ways to maintain my practice, especially in the context of managed care. For myself and many of my colleagues in a solo private practice, this has become a nightmare with entangled paperwork and never being sure of payment. This has made life more problematic and anxiety-provoking. This has also affected the hospitals where I work and has created uncertainty in many of the health professions. The future depends on adapting to these changes and using different skills to negotiate new expectations."

How Gerald D. Oster Got Started

"My initial undergraduate years from 1967 to 1971 was a time of social change and activism, and self-exploration. Although I began as a business major, the courses in sociology were much more appealing and the people's thinking in those courses were more similar to my viewpoints at the time.

"The prospect of studying topics such as social and political theory and how people adapt to environmental and economic change was very appealing. And the prospect of studying these topics on a higher level was challenging—that is, taking school and studying seriously, both on an undergraduate and graduate level.

"Also, learning about and helping people in all aspects of life filled a need in myself to go beyond my own boundaries and provide support to people in stress or to help the broader institutions in gaining the appropriate placement for people who needed assistance, whether it was the aged, juvenile delinquents, or children with learning problems.

"It was not until several years after receiving my undergraduate degree (and owning a bookstore for several years) that I was able to crystallize my thoughts into a single direction. I am sure this waiting is not unique. Only a few have a specific direction regarding careers and most go through college with the hope that the degree and higher education will get them some kind of a job. However, a career choice means much more. It is something that you know that you love and want to pursue full-time; in essence it becomes a paid hobby.

"For me, psychology was that path. And even in psychology, there were many roads to pursue. At first, I wanted to be a criminal psychologist and found courses in personality and psychopathology very fascinating. I also found courses in child development extremely interesting and had an outstanding professor that was able to demonstrate the early cognitive and emotional stages of life. My first choice, criminal psychology, took me to my first graduate school and my master's degree and to actual work within the juvenile justice system, providing evaluations for the courts on delinquents. However, through the support of my professors and continuing interest in all of psychology, I applied and was able to get into a doctoral program where I was exposed to a greater depth and breadth of psychology.

"While there, I worked in a rat laboratory, was part of a developing center for aging, taught courses in developmental psychology and child development, and was exposed to continuing clinical work through practicums at child development centers and psychiatric units for the aged. I also participated with many research teams on topics of learning theory, intellectual testing, and cognitive changes over the life span.

"I started my professional career in 1981 at a private research firm that subcontracted work from NIH. At the time, I was involved coordinating research projects for a nationwide study on depression. After a year, I decided to return to clinical work and obtained a job in a state hospital as a psychologist on an adolescent unit. During that time, I also consulted to a geriatric unit and continued my learning through weekly seminars and clinical rounds.

"After several years and having obtained my independent professional license I changed locations and jobs. I began working at a residential treatment center for emotionally disturbed children and adolescents. While there I became Director of Psychology Internship Training. I also continued my own training, which included study in family therapy at a well-known institute. I then became interested in expanding my private practice and continuing my writing, which I had begun during this time. So, I resigned and began collecting a series of part-time jobs.

"As far as my writing, I have now coauthored six professional books on psychological testing and therapy. I have also cowritten a trade book, entitled *Helping Your Depressed Teenager: A Guide for Parents and Caregivers* (Wiley, 1995). My latest book is *Clinical Uses of Drawings* (Jason Aronson, 1996)."

Expert Advice

"Learning is a lifelong process. Degrees only give you permission to learn. These were words from an uncle and ring true in today's world. Most people anticipate change and you can expect to change career paths several times during a lifetime. Thus, going to college and possibly to graduate school allows you this exposure to not only the gathering of technical skills, but also to possibilities. Even a field such as psychology has numerous outlets to pursue. In research there is test development, treatment outcomes, human factors studies, to name a few. In clinical you can work in hospitals, outpatient centers, residential treatment, and with various populations, such as infants, parent training, teenagers, adults with serious mental illness, or support to the healthy aged. Organizational psychologists work in work settings to devise screening tests or support the emotional needs of the staff or do staff development seminars. And psychologists teach courses in developmental or social issues, learning theory or cognitive-behavioral therapy, or other related topics.

"Along the way, you can define yourself in many ways. What it takes is sticking to a broad path and having the realization that the path may have many branches that are all quite good. But it takes exposure to these branches to realize the possibilities. So look around, read articles from journals or magazines by people who are doing the kind of work you can see yourself doing. And find out what is exciting and meaningful to you. Don't be afraid to talk to these people (they are human and approachable). If not them, talk to your professors; they want to help and have placed themselves as models and as valuable resources.

"Gain experience wherever you can, through paid or volunteer work. Go to seminars and to conventions, even if these are supposed to be for professionals. There is no better place to see the kinds of possibilities than at a national convention within a profession. You gain incredible exposure and an awareness of what the field is all about. Discovering your life's pursuit, something that you really love, is especially important, especially in the context of family.

"Also, gain mentors along the way. Become assistants, whether it is in teaching or research. This is an excellent way to discover what your strengths and weaknesses are, and whether you could see yourself doing this work on a daily basis. Take as many practicums or internships as possible.

"And travel. In striving for an ideal picture of yourself, you also want to be aware of possible settings. Do you enjoy the outdoors or city life? Does your profession offer more possibilities in small towns, where you actually perform more duties, than in large cities, where there are many specialists but more people, job opportunities, etc. What type of atmosphere do you prefer; the pressure of the Northeast or the slower pace of the South or alternative lifestyles of the Southwest."

● ● ●

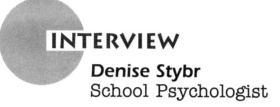

INTERVIEW
Denise Stybr
School Psychologist

Denise Stybr has been a school psychologist with the Center Cass School District #66 in Downers Grove, Illinois, since 1990. In 1979 she earned a B.S. in psychology from the University of Illinois, Urbana. Her M.A. in school psychology is from Governors State University in Illinois. She began her professional career in 1982.

What the Job's Really Like

"I administer psycho-educational testing to determine the presence or absence of a handicapping condition, such as a learning disability, mental retardation, or emotional disorder. I also provide individual and group counseling to the students, consultation to the parents and staff, and design behavior management programs.

"My job is extremely stressful, but never boring. I make life-changing decisions that affect both children and their families. From the moment I get to work, generally 7:30 A.M., until the moment I leave, generally 4:30 P.M., I am on. I am often met in the parking lot with questions and concerns. It is common for me to work the whole day with only a half an hour break at lunch. A typical day finds me attending several meetings at which we are usually deciding if a child should be tested and if he or she qualifies for services after the tests have been completed. Or I'm presenting the test results to the child's parents.

"In between meetings I usually hold two to three counseling sessions, spend two to three hours testing, and the remainder of the time writing reports, talking to teachers, or talking to parents. I travel to three schools, often within the same day. The office space I'm allocated ranges from very nice to nonexistent.

"I do not like the stress level or the all-too-often feeling that no matter what I do it isn't going to be enough for this child. But I do like the freedom and variety of my job. I rarely have to do any one thing at a specific time (with the exception of meetings). I can choose when to do what. I have control over my time."

How Denise Stybr Got Started

"I originally had thought to become a psychiatrist, but decided that medical school was not for me by my junior year in college. I then researched the different areas of graduate study for psychology and liked the freedom of school psychology. I do not have to maintain my own office or records. I do not have to purchase malpractice insurance for myself. I do not have to get coverage to go on a vacation. I never have to turn someone down who needs help but can't pay. (It's a free service through the schools.) And I mainly work with children age 3 to 14. In this age range lots of progress is still relatively easy to make.

"In order to practice as a certified school psychologist you must also complete a one-school-year internship, during which time you act as a school psychologist but are closely supervised by a certified school psychologist. In addition, 75 contact hours of continuing educational activities must be completed and documented every three years in order to continue to be nationally certificated.

"The reason I have a B.S. instead of a B.A. is that I originally was intent on medical school so I took more science courses than required for a B.A. My M.S. is a special kind of masters. In fact, it is often called a specialist degree because it requires 57 or more hours versus a regular masters that usually requires 30 to 32 hours."

Expert Advice

"Being a school psychologist requires a certain personality type, almost more than it does any special talent. One must be structured and organized, yet flexible. One must know when to take a stand and when to back down. You have to have empathy, but not sympathy, and compassion without sentimentality. A school psychologist often works with no peer input and must remain impartial.

"Seek after-school and summer jobs that put you around children and their parents. If possible volunteer with developmentally disabled children in order to see if you have what it takes to work with that population. Ask to observe in some special education classrooms.

"Don't expect to make a lot of money. School psychologists are often paid less than teachers. Benefits are often not as good as the teachers' contracts. Days are longer. We often work days during the summer that the teachers do not—generally a week or two before school starts and after school ends. This is not an easy, high-paying job. It is truly a vocation more than an occupation."

● ● ●

FOR MORE INFORMATION

For information on careers, educational requirements, financial assistance, and licensing in all fields of psychology, contact:

American Psychological Association
Education in Psychology and Accreditation Offices
Education Directorate
750 1st Street NE
Washington, DC 20002

For information on careers, educational requirements, and licensing of school psychologists, contact:

National Association of School Psychologists
8455 Colesville Road, Suite 1000
Silver Spring, MD 20910

Information about state licensing requirements is available from:

Association of State and Provincial Psychology Boards
P.O. Box 4389
Montgomery, AL 36103

Information on traineeships and fellowships also is available from colleges and universities that have graduate departments of psychology.

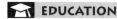

CHAPTER 7 **Psychiatrists**

EDUCATION
Postgraduate Required
Other

$$$ SALARY/EARNINGS
$60,000 to $100,000+

OVERVIEW

Medical doctors, or physicians as they are also known, examine patients; obtain medical histories; order, perform, and interpret diagnostic tests; and treat injuries, illnesses, and disorders. They also consult with other physicians, and if they are in private practice, take care of the business aspects of running an office.

Psychiatry is one of the many areas in which M.D.s can specialize. According to the American Medical Association, 6.3 percent of all doctors are psychiatrists. Psychiatrists can also specialize, in child psychiatry, for example, or geriatrics or neuropsychology.

Psychiatrists usually work with patients who suffer from any one of a number of mental illnesses. The main difference between psychiatrists and psychologists (see Chapter 1) is that M.D.s are able to prescribe medication. Psychiatrists utilize that privilege by prescribing a variety of drugs known to be effective in treating the various forms of mental illness.

About two out of three doctors have an office-based practice or work in clinics or HMOs; about one-fifth of all doctors are employed by hospitals. Others work for the federal government in veterans' hospitals, or for the Public Health Service in the Department of Health and Human Services.

Training for doctors is long and arduous, and once licensed and in practice the load doesn't decrease. Doctors have irregular schedules, and often work between 50 and 60 hours a week.

While traditionally doctors have always been solo practitioners, it is becoming more and more common to see partnerships or group practices. This arrangement allows doctors to be able to afford expensive equipment and enjoy other business advantages.

TRAINING

Most students enter medical school, which takes four years of study, with a bachelor's degree or even higher, then go on to do a residency.

Premedical studies include undergraduate work in biology, physics, and organic and inorganic chemistry.

The first two years of medical school include course work in anatomy, biochemistry, physiology, microbiology, pathology, medical ethics, and laws governing medicine.

During the last two years, students work under the supervision of experienced physicians learning acute, chronic, preventive, and rehabilitative care. Through rotations in family practice, internal medicine, obstetrics and gynecology, pediatrics, psychiatry, and surgery, medical students gain experience working directly with patients, diagnosing and treating illnesses.

After medical school, and after passing an examination given by the National Board of Medical Examiners, almost all new M.D.s go on to do a residency. The residency can take up to seven years depending upon the specialty they are pursuing. A subspecialty might require an additional one to two years of residency. After the residency is completed, doctors sit for a final examination given by The American Board of Medical Specialists. This is required for board certification.

JOB OUTLOOK

Employment of physicians is expected to grow faster than the average for all occupations through the year 2005 due to continued expansion of the health industry. New technologies permit more intensive care: physicians can do more tests, perform more procedures, and treat conditions previously regarded as untreatable. In addition, the population is growing and aging, and health care needs increase sharply with age. The need to replace physicians is lower than for most occupations because almost all physicians remain in the profession until they retire.

Job prospects are good for primary care physicians such as family practitioners and internists, and for geriatric and preventive care specialists.

Some shortages have been reported in the specialty areas of general surgery and psychiatry, and in some rural and low-income areas. This is because physicians find these areas unattractive due to low earnings potential, isolation from medical colleagues, or other reasons, not because of any overall shortage.

Some health care analysts believe that there is, or that there soon could be, a general oversupply of physicians; others disagree. In analyzing job prospects, it should be kept in mind that an oversupply may not necessarily limit the ability of physicians to find employment or to set up and maintain a practice. It could result in physicians performing more procedures than otherwise and delegating fewer tasks, or it could result in their providing more time to each patient, giving more attention to preventive care, and providing more services in rural and poor areas.

It is also possible that where surpluses are due to specialty imbalances, physicians in surplus specialties would provide services outside of their specialty area.

Unlike their predecessors, newly trained physicians face radically different choices of where and how to practice. Many new physicians are likely to avoid solo practice and take salaried jobs in group medical practices, clinics, and HMOs in order to have regular work hours and the opportunity for peer consultation.

Others will take salaried positions simply because they cannot afford the high costs of establishing a private practice while paying off student loans.

SALARIES

Earnings vary according to specialty; the number of years in practice; geographic region; hours worked; and skill, personality, and professional reputation.

According to the AMA (American Medical Association), average salaries after expenses ran about $120,000 a year in 1993.

But these are just averages. Some well-run office practices can pull in $500,000 a year or more. To offset this, it is important to remember that most doctors in private practice outlay a considerable sum of money for equipment and insurance and most new doctors have astronomical medical school loans to pay off.

RELATED FIELDS

Psychiatrists work to prevent, diagnose, and treat mental illnesses. Professionals in other occupations that require similar kinds of skill and critical judgment include psychologists, counselors, and therapists.

● ● ●

INTERVIEW
Gerald Horne
Psychiatrist

Gerald Horne became an M.D. in 1974. After three years of postgraduate training in psychiatry, he set up his own practice. He is also director of an inpatient, short-term psychiatric unit in a private suburban hospital.

What the Job's Really Like

"Because I can't get all the paperwork done during the day, when I finish the evening hours, instead of staying around in the office dictating, I bring the charts home. A typical day starts with me getting up in the morning around 5:30, quarter to 6:00, and I'll dictate the remaining charts, for whatever amount of time it takes; it could be half an hour or 45 minutes. Then I'll go to the hospital and make rounds. These are patients who have been hospitalized for all sorts of psychiatric problems, such as depression or schizophrenia. The majority of our patients are teenagers, although we admit adults and geriatric patients too.

"I have a team of psychiatric RNs, mental health counselors, and social workers I supervise. I always try to finish my rounds on time so I can be available for consultations with the staff and to lead the first group therapy session of the day, which usually begins around 9:00.

"We have a team approach to therapy on our unit. A patient is assigned to a particular staff member, but several might sit in on individual therapy sessions and contribute to the treatment plan. We also try to involve the families, and we schedule those meetings throughout the day.

"In the late afternoon and sometimes in the evening I see private patients in an office I have in a group practice.

"The real benefit to my job, to psychiatry, is being able to develop a continuing relationship with the patient and the patient's family—and seeing them learn how to deal with the problems they have. That's very important and very rewarding to me.

"There are a bunch of negative aspects. Government intervention is one. And I don't enjoy the copious paperwork I have to deal with.

"The other consideration is the malpractice problem. It's a very litigious society and everybody is out to lay their suit. So you're constantly making sure that you're dotting that 'i' and crossing that 't' and documenting everything you can into the chart. You don't want someone to come back at you one day and try to level a suit at you. That's an unpleasant part of medicine.

"But the most pleasant part is that I think the practice of psychiatry is not pure science; it's both art and science. And that makes life more enjoyable."

How Gerald Horne Got Started

"It goes way, way back to a nice Jewish mother who put a lot of emphasis on the professions. That was a major factor as a starting point. I also knew that whatever I ended up doing, I wanted to be independent, to be in charge of my life and not have to answer to anybody. And when I say that, I mean that I have my own practice, I run the office myself, the way I feel it needs to be run. I don't have to worry about having a boss, punching a time card, or being fired at a moment's notice. But things have changed through the years and they've changed tremendously. In the old days you ran a very independent practice, with, but separate from, Medicare and private insurances and you could do as you saw fit. But now we have to jump through many hoops. It is becoming more and more regulated and that's a problem now, and not why I went into medicine.

"Another component of why I chose this profession was that I wanted to be able to work with people, because I feel I have a lot of empathy. And the final component was that the profession is challenging.

"When I started medical school I had wanted to be a pediatrician. I was very interested in working with children. During medical school you rotate through all the different specialties, internal medicine, ob/gyn, surgery, pediatrics, family medicine. And lo and behold I finished the first year and I found out there were big people, too. I discovered I really liked the concept of being able to deal with the entire family too."

Expert Advice

"Getting into medical school is exceedingly difficult. It doesn't really make sense, but with more government regulations and more problems in medicine than ever before, we're getting more applicants than ever before. Probably the most important thing for a student considering a premed course is that the first year in college is most important. Freshman year students are often feeling their oats and enjoying their liberties and might not be studying quite as much as they should. If, by the time the second year rolls around, they decide they really want to go into medicine, but their first year was not very successful, it can really drag them down. Have fun, enjoy yourself, but really try to concentrate on academics and not get behind in your work. If you start out with a low GPA, it's almost impossible to catch up."

● ● ●

FOR MORE INFORMATION

For a list of medical schools and general information on training, financial aid, and medicine as a career contact:

The American Medical Association (AMA)
515 North State Street
Chicago, IL 60610

Association of American Medical Colleges
Section for Student Services
2450 N Street, NW
Washington, DC 20037-1131.

For information on osteopathic medicine as a career contact:

American Osteopathic Association
Department of Public Relations
142 East Ontario Street
Chicago, IL 60611

American Association of Colleges of Osteopathic Medicine
6110 Executive Boulevard, Suite 405
Rockville, MD 20852

CHAPTER 8 Psychiatric Nurses

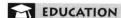 **EDUCATION**

B.A./B.S. Preferred
Other

$$$ SALARY/EARNINGS

$20,000 to $53,000

OVERVIEW

Although you don't have to have an R.N. to find a satisfying career in the helping professions, most nurses feel they can better help people by taking into account both physical and emotional factors.

Registered psychiatric nurses can work with very emotionally disturbed patients or with patients who are basically well and just need support with normal problems. In order to make the right career choice, it is important to understand the type of work you would be doing. In a hospital setting you would deal with all types of patients. Many of them could be chronically ill without much hope for improvement. They could be severely depressed, suicidal, or violent and not be able to function in normal lives.

Generally, in mental health clinics or health centers, patients will have less severe problems and the opportunities to help and see improvement are greater. You might work with clients going through a divorce or grieving over the loss of a child or a spouse.

Approximately 68 percent of all nurses work in hospital settings. Others work in clinics, private doctors' offices, nursing homes, training rooms, first aid stations at sporting events, summer camps, school infirmaries, rehabilitation centers, outpatient centers, and even prisons. They work in rural areas, such as on Indian reservations, in Alaska, or in the Appalachian Mountains, or around the world on cruise ships, with the Armed Forces, the Foreign Service, the Peace Corps, or the Red Cross. Some also, in much the same way a doctor does, set up their own office and work in private practice. Others even make home visits.

Working conditions vary depending upon the setting. RNs in a psychiatric hospital are usually paid on the same scale as floor nurses in other departments. Nurses working in health centers or clinics are generally paid more.

Hospital nurses often work more erratic hours—they can be scheduled for holidays, weekends, nights, evenings, and days. Nurses in a clinic generally have the benefit of more normal hours, Monday through Friday with only an occasional evening or weekend.

Hospital settings more typically follow a "medical model," viewing the people they're helping as "patients" who are sick, relying on medication as a large segment of the therapy process.

Therapists in clinics view the people they are helping as basically well. Here they are called "clients." Therapy is usually more active, relying on talking, support, and education, working toward specific, achievable goals.

TRAINING

To obtain a nursing license, all states require graduation from an accredited nursing school and passing a national licensing examination. Nurses may be licensed in more than one state, either by examination or endorsement of a license issued by another state. Licenses must be periodically renewed, and continuing education is a requirement for renewal in some states.

In 1993, there were 1,493 entry-level R.N. programs. At present, there are four different ways you can become a registered nurse:

1. Through a two-year community college, earning an associate's degree (A.D.N.) in nursing

2. Through a three-year hospital-based nursing school, earning a diploma

3. Through a four- or five-year university program, resulting in the Bachelor's of Science degree in nursing, or the B.S.N., as it is commonly called

4. For those who already have a bachelor's degree in a different subject, there is a "generic" master's degree in nursing, a two- to three-year program beyond the bachelor's degree.

More than 60 percent of graduates in 1993 were from A.D.N. programs. More than one-quarter of graduates in 1993 were from diploma and B.S.N. programs.

Generally, licensed graduates of any of the three program types qualify for entry-level positions as staff nurses.

There have been attempts to raise the educational requirements for an R.N. license to a bachelor's degree and, possibly, create new job titles. However, such proposals have been around for years.

These changes, should they occur, will be made state by state, through legislation or regulation. Changes in licensure requirements would not affect currently licensed R.N.s, who would be grandfathered in, no matter what their educational preparation.

However, individuals considering nursing should carefully weigh the pros and cons of enrolling in a B.S.N. program, since advancement opportunities are broader for those with a B.S.N. In fact, some career paths are open only to nurses with bachelor's or advanced degrees.

While A.D.N. or diploma preparation is enough for a nursing home nurse to advance to director of nursing, a bachelor's degree is generally necessary for administrative positions in hospitals and for positions in community nursing. Moreover, the B.S.N. is a prerequisite for admission to graduate nursing programs. So individuals considering positions requiring graduate training, such as research, consulting, teaching, or clinical specializations, should enroll in a B.S.N. program.

A growing number of A.D.N. and diploma-trained nurses are entering bachelor's programs to prepare for a broader scope of nursing practice. They can often find a hospital position and then take advantage of tuition reimbursement programs to get a B.S.N.

For many nursing specialties, it is essential to also earn a master's degree or an advanced certificate; and for some nurses, those who wish to teach, for example, a Ph.D., or doctorate, in nursing is required.

To specialize in psychiatric nursing, you would need an R.N. as a minimum, and then your B.S.N. Some settings require further education and you could study for a master's degree in counseling, psychiatric nursing, clinical psychology, or social work.

Nursing education includes classroom instruction and supervised training in hospitals and other health facilities. Students take courses in anatomy, physiology, microbiology, chemistry, nutrition, psychology and other behavioral sciences, and nursing.

Supervised clinical experience is provided in hospital departments such as pediatrics, psychiatry, maternity, and surgery. A growing number of programs include courses in gerontological nursing and clinical practice in nursing homes. Some provide clinical training in public health departments and home health agencies.

Nurses should be caring and sympathetic. They must be able to accept responsibility, direct or supervise others, follow orders precisely, and determine when consultation is required.

Experience and good performance can lead to promotion to increasingly more responsible positions. Nurses can advance, in management, to assistant head nurse or head nurse. From there, they can advance to assistant director, director, and vice president positions. Increasingly, management-level nursing positions require a graduate degree in nursing or health services administration. They also require leadership, negotiation skills, and good judgment. Graduate programs preparing executive-level nurses usually last one to two years.

JOB OUTLOOK

Job prospects in nursing are good. Although employers in some parts of the country reported shortages of RNs in the past, large wage increases have attracted more people to nursing and dampened demand. However, RN recruitment has long been a problem in rural areas, in some big city hospitals, and in specialty areas including intensive care, rehabilitation, geriatrics, and long-term care.

Employment of registered nurses is expected to grow much faster than the average for all occupations through the year 2005. Driving this growth will be technological advances in patient care, which permit a greater number of medical problems to be treated, and increasing emphasis on primary care.

Many job openings will result from the need to replace experienced nurses who leave the occupation, especially as the average age of the registered nurse population continues to rise.

Employment in hospitals, the largest sector, is expected to grow more slowly than in other health care sectors. While the intensity of nursing care is likely to increase, requiring more nurses per patient, the number of inpatients is not likely to increase much.

Most rapid growth is expected in hospitals' outpatient facilities.

Employment in private practices and clinics, including HMOs, and emergency medical centers is expected to grow very rapidly as health care in general expands.

SALARIES

Median weekly earnings of full-time salaried registered nurses were $682 in 1994. The middle 50 percent earned between $542 and $838. The lowest 10 percent earned less than $395; the top 10 percent, more than $1,005.

According to a University of Texas Medical Branch survey of hospitals and medical centers, the median annual salary of staff nurses, based on a 40-hour week and excluding shift or area differentials, was $35,256 in October 1994. The average minimum salary was $28,531 and the average maximum was $43,711. For head nurses, the median was $50,700.

Many employers are offering flexible work schedules, child care, educational benefits, bonuses, and other incentives.

RELATED FIELDS

Workers in other occupations with responsibilities and duties similar to those of registered psychiatric nurses are mental health counselors, rehab counselors, and social workers.

INTERVIEW

Monica James
Counselor/Nurse

Monica James has been a nurse for 10 years and a counselor/educator at a women's health center for five. Last year she became director of the center. She recently finished work on her master's degree in clinical psychology.

What the Job's Really Like

"Our clinic is a department of a small community hospital. We're wellness-oriented in that we deal mainly with a population of well women. We try to meet our client's health information needs and address their emotional well-being. We offer a lot of different support groups. They're basically designed for women because men don't often come to them. We have support groups for women who have had breast cancer, we have all kinds of bereavement groups such as for widows, or for parents who have lost a child, or adults who have lost a parent. We also have a weekly domestic violence support and education group for women. By giving them support and information we help empower women.

"We also run workshops on self-esteem, relationship skills, communication skills, assertiveness training, parenting, and adjustment to divorce. Our clients are mostly working and professional women, 35 to 55 years old.

"In the morning I might have a few one-on-one counseling sessions with clients, covering divorce or self-esteem issues. Then there's the administrative duties, the paperwork. And I coordinate with other health care professionals and make referrals for my clients.

"I also sometimes give presentations in the community for a women's organization or a business. Right now I'm working on a workshop for the postal service on managing anger. It's called 'The Anger in You.'

"In the afternoon I attend a meeting or two, then work on our newsletter, which we distribute to our clients. I have to read a lot, too. There's always a lot of new information coming into the clinic and I have to keep informed.

"What I like most is getting to work with women who are basically well. Sometimes in a hospital setting you can feel as if your efforts are not showing results, but in this kind of job you can feel you're making a difference. You can see your clients getting their needs met.

"I also like the idea of being independent. In my field you can collaborate with other professionals but you're not given a prescribed way of doing things. I can be very creative.

"In fact, I like everything about my job. I can't think of even one negative."

How Monica James Got Started

"Twelve years ago when I started my training, I had this vision of myself in a starched white uniform, handing glasses of water to patients with their medications, smiling, and brightening their day. Boy was I naive then. Through the training program I had a chance to see all sorts of nursing situations. I learned pretty early on that I preferred working not in a hospital setting. I wanted to work with well people, not the chronically ill.

"The university I attended had a hospital and a counseling center and it's there I realized that I could use my nurse's training and counseling skills to treat the whole person.

"I started off a counselor/educator, then went back for my master's degree. I was promoted to assistant director, then when the director left, I was offered the position—and gladly took it."

Expert Advice

"You can start off by getting involved in any peer counseling programs your school might offer. Later, you can volunteer and then find part-time work in a variety of mental health settings. During this process you will get a feel for what the work is really like and you will be able to make an informed choice. You will also learn how to assess yourself and to see if you have what it takes."

●　●　●

INTERVIEW

Rob Verner
Psychiatric Nurse

Rob Verner has been a psychiatric nurse for more than 15 years. He works in an inpatient hospital setting.

What the Job's Really Like

"I work on three different units in my hospital. There's a psychiatric emergency room, from where most of our patients are admitted, a short-term acute psychiatric unit for agitated patients, and a unit for adolescents age 10 to 18.

"Some of the patients are very depressed, even suicidal. Others suffer from schizophrenia and hear voices or see things that aren't there. Some of the patients are violent. I can put on the nightly news before I come into work and hear about how the police apprehended a man waving a gun on the street. I know that when I get to work, he'll be there waiting for me.

"The adolescents we get have severe problems at home or at school or they're depressed or suicidal. Occasionally, we get an early schizophrenic who is starting to hear voices. That's very sad.

"On a typical day, I start by getting the report from the last shift and find out what was happening on the unit while I was off. Then I greet all the patients I am assigned to and tell them who I am and that I'll be taking care of them. I discuss with them any special activities going on, with the recreational therapist or occupational therapist, for example.

"Later in the day I hand out medications, then talk with each patient about why they're in the hospital and how they're feeling.

"I also spend a lot of time setting limits and 'redirecting,' trying to control behavior. A lot of the time I find myself saying things like, 'You can't go into that other patient's room, you need to stay in your own room or in the day room; you can't threaten to hit that person because you're angry with him; you have to put that chair down and not hit anybody with it.' It's an acute unit and we have some violent patients.

"I also teach patients about their medications, and help them look for alternative ways to deal with their problems. Then there's the administrative duties, charting on the patients or attending meetings with the psychiatrists, social workers, and various therapists to discuss care plans.

"I like having a lot of contact with just a few patients. I could have gone into psychology or even psychiatry if I had wanted to, but I think in those fields you see an awful lot of patients for a brief period of time during the week. What I am attracted to is spending a lot of time with fewer patients.

"But the job is very emotionally stressful, the violence and the behavioral problems. And it's hard dealing with other people's problems; you can lose the energy to deal with your own problems.

"The hours can be very difficult, too, when you're rotating shifts, working nights, evenings, working days. You can get confused as to what day it is.

"And sometimes it's stressful dealing with the doctors. You might have different ideas how a patient should be treated and you can spend a lot of time trying to get ahold of the doctor for medication orders, etc. Generally, in psychiatric nursing, you don't get to use your own brain sometimes. You know what the patient needs, but you can't do anything until you get ahold of the physician. Having your actions limited is frustrating.

"It's also frustrating dealing with the chronically ill. You can't cure anybody, can't make the disease go away."

How Rob Verner Got Started

"When I was in college I had a work-study job at a state mental hospital. After I got out of college with my liberal arts degree I wasn't sure what I wanted to do. I looked at all the jobs I'd had in my life and the one I liked the most was at the hospital. So I went and got another job similar to that one, but the pay was terrible. Someone suggested I become a nurse and I laughed. I had never considered it before. But then I thought about it some more and asked myself why not. So I did it.

"I already had a bachelor's degree, in general studies, but there was a program at Case Western Reserve for people just like me. I studied for 23 months straight and earned my B.S.N."

Expert Advice

"The few people you can really help makes it all worthwhile, but you have to be prepared for all the people you can't help. If you're the type of person who gets stressed out easily, then this setting might not be for you. There are plenty of easier settings for psychiatric nursing—clinics, for one. In a hospital you see a lot of chronic patients—and you have to be ready to deal with shift work."

● ● ●

FOR MORE INFORMATION

The National League for Nursing (NLN) publishes a variety of nursing and nursing education materials, including a list of nursing schools and information on student financial aid. For a complete list of NLN publications, write for a career information brochure. Send your request to:

Communications Department
National League for Nursing
350 Hudson Street
New York, NY 10014

For a list of B.S.N. and graduate programs, write to:

American Association of Colleges of Nursing
1 Dupont Circle, Suite 530
Washington, DC 20036

Information on career opportunities as a registered nurse is available from:

American Nurses' Association
600 Maryland Avenue SW
Washington, DC 20024-2571

Society for Education and Research in Psychiatric-Mental Health Nursing
437 Twin Bay Drive
Pensacola, FL 32534

Information about employment opportunities in Department of Veterans Affairs medical centers is available from local VA medical centers and also from:

Title 38 Employment Division (054D)
Department of Veterans Affairs
810 Vermont Avenue NW
Washington, DC 20420

For information on child psychiatric nursing careers write to:

Advocates for Child Psychiatric Nursing
437 Twin Bay Drive
Pensacola, FL 32534

CHAPTER 9

Physical and Occupational Therapists

 EDUCATION

B.A./B.S. Required
Postgraduate Preferred
Other

$$$ SALARY/EARNINGS

$20,000 to $45,000

OVERVIEW

Physical and occupational therapists help people with physical and emotional limitations to reach their full potential.

The purpose of physical therapy is to correct muscular-skeletal dysfunction and problems with movement. The physical therapist works pretty independently, evaluating patients, designing and implementing treatment plans.

The American Occupational Therapy Association defines occupational therapy as "a health and rehabilitation profession. Its practitioners provide services to individuals of all ages who have physical, developmental, emotional, and social deficits, and because of these conditions, need specialized assistance in learning skills to enable them to lead independent, productive, and satisfying lives."

The Differences Between PTs and OTs

PTs and OTs differ from each other in a few ways. Although they have the same goals, to make the patient as independent as possible, physical therapists deal with only the patients' physical difficulties. OTs work with physical and psychosocial aspects. A lot of occupational therapists work in psychiatric facilities, helping patients to cope with their emotional problems. And some patients have a combination of problems. They might have had a stroke, but are suffering from depression as well.

And while they both deal with physical problems, they don't do it in the same way. An occupational therapist probably wouldn't help a person with ambulation skills, learning how to walk. However, both the physical and occupational therapist might focus on transfer skills, helping a person get from the bed to a chair, from the chair to a standing position.

SETTINGS FOR PHYSICAL THERAPISTS

While those not in the know might think of physical therapists as working only in hospital setting, there is, in actuality, a wide range of settings open to PT professionals. In addition to seeing patients in acute-care hospitals, both inpatient and outpatient, physical therapists see patients in their homes, providing home health care; in schools, working with students on the playing fields; in nursing homes; in rehab hospitals; in private practices; and in industry, doing job-site analyses, helping to prevent injuries. As an example, IBM or another large corporation could hire a physical therapist to evaluate risks the employees encounter, and then by following the recommendations made by the physical therapist, they can redesign the workplace and lower their workers' compensation payments.

Physical therapists can also travel, working for what is called a traveling company. This kind of company will make sure you are licensed in whatever state you might go to, and then they will send you around the country on temporary assignments, wherever there is a need.

Physical therapists work with the following patients or problems:

Premature infants

Pediatric patients

Obstetric patients

People with sports or traumatic injuries

People with birth or genetic defects

Adults with back or neck injuries

Stroke victims

Burn and wound victims

Amputees

Dancers and performing artists

Athletes

People with muscular sclerosis, Parkinson's disease, or neurological injuries

Postoperative patients

Geriatric patients

TRAINING FOR PHYSICAL THERAPISTS

Physical therapists must have at least a bachelor's degree. Some go on for a master's and others earn their doctorate. Most schools require anywhere from 20 to 100 hours of observation time before future PTs can even apply to be admitted to a program. This observation time can be clocked while volunteering or working as a physical therapy aide.

Physical therapy programs can be found through the American Physical Therapy Association, whose address is listed at the end of this chapter.

Coursework covers mostly math and sciences as well as specific training on the techniques used in physical therapy, including exercise science and exercise physiology. Although the training is similar to that undertaken by personal trainers (the personal trainer occupation is covered in *On the Job: Real People Providing Services*), physical therapy training is more medically based. PT students study more pathology, doing cadaver dissections, for example. The study of anatomy and physiology is more extensive, as is muscle pathology. But the differences are explained easily by the different people each works with. Personal trainers deal with a healthy population for the most part; physical therapists work with patients who have disabilities or a variety of other problems mentioned above.

Physical Therapist Assistant

While the physical therapist is responsible for the design of treatment plans, the physical therapist assistant is trained to carry out those plans. Limitations for the physical therapist assistant are that they cannot update or change treatment plans.

Training for a physical therapist assistant career involves a two-year program ending with an associate's degree.

Physical Therapy Aide

Physical therapy aides are usually trained on the job. They can't do direct patient care, but they help out the physical therapist and the physical therapist assistant. Aides might help a patient count the number of exercises he is doing, move equipment, bring patients to the treatment areas, or help a person walk or transfer from the bed to a chair.

SALARIES FOR THE PHYSICAL THERAPY PROFESSION

A brand new graduate physical therapist can make an excellent starting salary—between $35,000 to $40,000 a year, depending upon the region of the country in which he or she chooses to practice. Salaries go up with the number of years' experience.

Physical therapists working in home health can make $40 to $50 an hour, and physical therapists in private practice can make between $85,000 and $100,000 a year. But these self-employed physical therapists have more expenses to cover, too, such as insurance. In private practice, a physical therapist has to wear many hats, one of which is that of bill collector. And it can be difficult sometimes to collect payments owed you.

Traveling physical therapists usually make a good hourly salary and have all their expenses covered including flights, rental cars, hotel rooms, and meals.

Physical therapy assistants with a two-year degree can start out earning between $20,000 and $30,000 a year.

The nonprofessional position of physical therapy aide earns about $5 or so an hour.

JOB OUTLOOK FOR PHYSICAL THERAPISTS

The job outlook for physical therapists is excellent. There has been a shortage of physical therapists for quite a while now. There are two main reasons for this. The capabilities and problems that the physical therapist is qualified to handle have expanded, creating more of a demand.

Second, because academia doesn't pay well, there is a shortage of qualified people willing to teach in physical therapy training programs. When the teacher makes less money than the student, there is little motivation to follow that career path. Physical therapists with doctorates are required to teach master's and doctoral level students. Those numbers of qualified teachers are very low. Most physical therapists prefer to work in the field rather than in a classroom. With fewer teachers, fewer physical therapists can be trained, thus contributing to the shortage and increasing the demand.

SETTINGS FOR OCCUPATIONAL THERAPISTS

OTs work with all types of patients, from the premature infant to geriatric patients, and see people with all kinds of diagnoses. This covers anything that would limit their ability to care for themselves—arthritis, hand injuries, burns, and neurological dysfunction, which takes in stroke patients, patients with MS or muscular dystrophy, cerebral palsy, brain tumors, and psychiatric problems.

OTs work in the following settings:

Acute care hospitals

Rehab hospitals

Psychiatric hospitals or wards

Pediatric hospitals or wards

Nursing homes

School systems

Private practice

TRAINING FOR OCCUPATIONAL THERAPISTS

Occupational therapists must earn a four-year degree, studying all the sciences—zoology, biology, physiology, anatomy, kinesiology. You also take psychology and abnormal psychology classes as well as child development.

After your four years, you will do a six- to nine-month internship, rotating in different kinds of facilities and specialties.

Once you pass your internship, you have to take a national exam to become a registered occupational therapist.

Specialties you can study are pediatrics, psychiatric, hands, and physical disabilities.

Some OTs go on for master's degrees in occupational therapy or related fields such as administration or even physical therapy.

The personality qualities and skills you'll need to make a good OT are as follows: You should be outgoing, with a lot of empathy and a good sense of humor. You'll need to be open and be willing to talk to your patients. You also have to be a good listener. Patients look at their therapists as someone they can talk to—doctors rarely have enough time for that kind of relationship. You also need good people skills, dealing with coworkers and the family members of your patients.

Certified Occupational Therapy Assistants

Certified occupational therapy assistants study at a community college and earn a two-year associate's degree. Although they don't evaluate patients or make treatment plans, they function much as physical therapy assistants do, carrying out the plans.

Some universities have started weekend programs for OT assistants who want to get their four-year degree. While they are employed full time, they study every other weekend, finishing the bachelor's degree in about two years.

Occupational Therapy Aides

Occupational therapy aides function similarly to their PT counterparts, helping the OTs and assistants with various duties.

SALARIES FOR THE OCCUPATIONAL THERAPY PROFESSION

Salaries for OTs are similar to those for physical therapists and can start at around an average of $35,000 a year. Starting salaries for certified occupational therapy assistants would average about $20,000 a year. Occupational therapy aides would earn from $5 to $5.50 an hour.

RELATED FIELDS

Others who work in the rehabilitation field include corrective therapists, recreational therapists, manual arts therapists, speech pathologists and audiologists, prosthetists, respiratory therapists, chiropractors, acupuncturists, and personal and athletic trainers.

INTERVIEW

Laurie DeJong
Physical Therapist

Laurie DeJong is assistant director of physical therapy at a large community hospital. She graduated in 1984 with a bachelor's degree in physical therapy from Quinnipiac College in Hamden, Connecticut.

What the Job's Really Like

"Physical therapists generally specialize, working in a particular setting or with certain kinds of patients. We evaluate patients, looking for pain, their flexibility or range of motion, their strength, and what kind of functional activities they do or need to do. For example, if the patient is a dancer, she needs to dance; if it's a child, she needs to play; if it's an adult, she needs to work, and so on. We do a complete evaluation, sitting down and talking to the patient about what the patient is looking for, about what we're looking for, and then, depending upon the person and his or her needs, we would design an appropriate treatment plan.

"Treatment plans generally include manual therapy, doing stretching or strengthening exercises, or specific joint mobilization exercises. We also use modalities such as hot packs, cold packs, ultrasound, or electric stimulation to help reduce pain.

"We do a lot of teaching, too, explaining the exercises to the patients, so they can carry on the activities at home without us. We do a lot of education in terms of posture and how patients can prevent their injuries from recurring. If our patients are children, we also work with the parents or teachers, how to do the exercises or how to best help the child function in the school arena. On the sports field we may be educating the coaches as to what kind of exercises a specific child needs.

"We also run classes, such as back schools, body awareness, or risk management, within the hospital and within industry.

"Part of the job is doing documentation—that's the part most of us don't like, but it's necessary.

"But it's a great profession to have. You can specialize in so many different areas. We all come out with a basic background and then you can tailor your expertise to the area you prefer.

"In my job I like the fact that I can do a lot of different things. We have a lot of hands-on time with our patients. We develop a treatment plan and then we see the patients generally two or three times a week for at least a month. I like working with the kids because I can see them for years. A child with developmental delays, such as cerebral palsy, for example, I'll see forever. We get to develop a rapport, spending time one-on-one with our patients. Doctor's don't have the time to do that.

"I also like being able to keep up with the changes in health care, keeping myself on the cutting edge of what's happening out there.

"The stresses are the same as for everyone else. There's not enough time to do the job you have to do. It's also a challenge with the changes that are happening in health care. Some of the changes aren't fun and we don't like what's happening. There are now insurance companies telling us how we should treat our patients, as opposed to our dictating the kind of care our patients need. You'll find patients saying they know they need more treatment, but they won't be coming back to you because they can't afford it."

How Laurie DeJong Got Started

"I spent four years working in a rehab hospital and while there I started doing pediatrics and spent two years working with children as well as adults on an outpatient basis.

"For one year I had my own private practice doing home health and consultation in schools. I then moved to another state and joined the hospital as a staff physical therapist.

"I always liked medical things. I started playing hospital when I was about two. My parents told me I couldn't be a nurse, but I could become a doctor if I wanted to. But when I was 17 I realized how long it would take me to become a doctor. I learned about physical therapy from a guidance counselor, then realized that it would be the right career for me."

Expert Advice

"You have to really love working with people and you have to possess a great deal of patience. Change and improvement don't happen overnight. Often the person you're working with is impatient to get better, but you have to be the steadying force."

• • •

INTERVIEW

Helen Cox
Occupational Therapist

Helen Cox is an occupational therapy supervisor in the Rehab Services Department of a community hospital.

What the Job's Really Like

"Occupational therapy is a health profession that helps people to do things for themselves within the limits of their disability or disease.

"First of all, we need to evaluate the patients to see what their skills are or where they have some deficits. Then we have to make a decision on whether we can improve those deficits. For instance, if someone has had a stroke, and he or she has a weak arm on the side of the stroke, do we feel we can, through exercise and other activities, improve the function of the arm and get it back to what it was prior to the stroke?

"We have to see if the person has the motor ability, the muscle power, the strength to perform any activities. Does he or she have the coordination? Sometimes a person might have the motor power but couldn't pick up a coin from the table. That means this person would be limited in doing some things for himself or herself.

"Sometimes in the evaluation, we realize that with arthritic patients, for example, they have lost the ability to manipulate small buttons. Then we can look into some adaptive equipment such as button hooks, dressing sticks, or elastic shoelaces, which don't need as fine a motor ability to use.

"After the assessment we set realistic goals with the patient. 'Where do you want to be functioning in a month? Where do you want to be functioning in three or four months?' The goals may be as simple as putting on socks or a sweater, or as long range as being able to sew or play the piano.

"When we have the goals, we use various activities, from putting round pegs in round holes to maybe even practicing the piano or using a computer keyboard. It depends on what skills the patient is trying to develop.

"At the end of 30 days we evaluate the progress. We may have initially measured grip and pinch strength and then we'll measure them again to see if there's been improvement.

"If we haven't reached the goals we look to see why. Maybe the patient had another stroke or something else interfered. If we do reach the goals, we make new short-term goals until the patient has reached his or her maximum potential.

"Being able to see people improve is the nicest part of the job. Sometimes patients surprise you with what they're able to accomplish."

How Helen Cox Got Started

"I originally planned to become a nurse, but while I was away at college, I was having problems with chemistry. My brother, who is a physical therapist, said to me, 'Why do you want to become a nurse, anyway, and work all those ridiculous hours on weekends, nights, and holidays?' My mom was a nurse and that's why I was pursuing it. My brother suggested I become an occupational therapist and I said, 'What's that?' He was working at a VA hospital, so I went there to visit the occupational therapy clinic. I saw that it was a lot of hands-on care and then I knew that that's what I wanted to do. I went to the University of Illinois in Chicago and earned my B.S. in occupational therapy in 1970."

Expert Advice

"A lot of people who think they want a career in the health professions consider becoming a doctor or a nurse the only options. But that couldn't be further from the truth. You need to understand what each area of the health professions does, then make your choice based on your own personality makeup."

• • •

FOR MORE INFORMATION

American College of Sports Medicine (ACSM)
Member and Chapter Services Department
P.O. Box 1440
Indianapolis, IN 46206
    (Provides certification for personal trainers)

American Council on Exercise (ACE)
P.O. Box 910449
San Diego, CA 92191
    (Provides certification for personal trainers)

American Occupational Therapy Association
P.O. Box 1725
1383 Piccard Drive
Rockville, MD 20849-1725

American Physical Therapy Association
1111 North Fairfax Street
Alexandria, VA 22314

American Therapeutic Recreation Association
c/o Associated Management Systems
P.O. Box 15215
Hattiesburg, MS 39402-5215

International Physical Fitness Association
415 West Court Street
Flint, MI 48503

National Council for Therapeutic Recreation Certification
P.O. Box 479
Thiells, NY 10984-0479

National Therapeutic Recreation Society
2775 South Quincy Street, Suite 300
Arlington, VA 22206-2204

CHAPTER 10 Speech-Language Pathologists and Audiologists

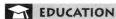 **EDUCATION**

Postgraduate Required
Other

$$$ SALARY/EARNINGS

$28,000 to $60,000

OVERVIEW

According to the American Speech-Language-Hearing Association (ASHA), speech and language disorders are "inabilities of individuals to understand and/or appropriately use the speech and language systems of society. Such disorders may range from simple sound repetitions or occasional miscalculations to the complete absence of the ability to use speech and language for communication."

For every 20 Americans who communicate "normally," there is one individual who is afflicted with a speech-language disorder. That numbers nearly 10 million people.

Hearing impairment ranges from the inability to hear speech and other sounds loudly enough and/or understand speech even when it is loud enough, to the complete loss of any hearing.

Based on studies of a decade ago by the National Center for Health Statistics, it is estimated that hearing impairment in one or both ears affects approximately 2 out of every 100 school-age children; 29 out of every 100 people 65 years of age or older; and a total of 21.2 million Americans.

A career as a speech-language pathologist or audiologist offers an opportunity to help and interact with a wide variety of individuals, providing rewarding experiences for both the client and therapist. It is also a career for the researcher dedicated to finding new therapeutic approaches and technology.

Speech-Language Pathology

A speech-language pathologist has a wide range of duties and choice of settings, age groups, and disorders with which to work. Speech-language pathologists screen, evaluate, and treat people with communication disorders. They also make referrals, provide counseling and instruction, supervise students and clinical fellows, teach, conduct research, and administer speech-language pathology programs.

Speech and language disorders can include:

- Disfluencies including stuttering and other interruptions of normal speech flow such as excessive hesitations, repeating the first sound in a word over and over, too frequently inserting extraneous syllables ("er," or "um,") or words and phrases into speech.

- Articulation disorders, substituting one sound for another ("free" instead of "three"), omitting a sound, or distorting a sound.

- Voice disorders, inappropriate pitch, quality, loudness, resonance, and duration.

- Aphasia, complete loss of speech (generally resulting from a stroke or head injury).

- Delayed language ability.

Those working in elementary schools spend a great deal of the time providing articulation therapy or phonologic therapy, teaching children to articulate more clearly. Some of the techniques they use involve playing games that have the child work with the same target sounds. Another technique is called auditory bombardment, and it uses a set of headphones that amplifies the therapist's speech and plays it into the child's ear. The therapist reads a list of words that are amplified, helping the child focus on the correct sounds.

Another interesting and unfortunately common disorder for speech-language pathologists to deal with is aphasia, an inability to either understand or produce speech due to a brain injury or brain disorder. This condition most commonly follows a stroke and sometimes follows brain trauma or accidents.

Although relying less heavily on devices than audiologists, speech-language pathologists do use equipment to check the health of vocal cords and detect any abnormal growths.

Audiology

The primary functions of audiologists are to test hearing and to do rehabilitation work with hearing-impaired individuals and their significant others.

To test hearing and the functioning of the auditory system, audiologists use a range of electronic equipment, the audiometer and other devices for assessing performance of hearing aids. There are devices that plug into hearing aids and can be programmed so that the performance of the hearing aid is appropriate for the hearing loss of that individual. There are also devices with very tiny microphones that are hooked up into tubes inserted directly into the ear canal to tell just how much sound is reaching the ear drum. Other devices test the functioning of a hearing aid independently of a person to make sure that all the electronics in the aid are working correctly.

The primary effect of a person's hearing loss is on the ability to communicate and the ability to hear speech. For most people, the most important person they want to be able to communicate with is their spouse or significant other. Therefore, therapy will focus not only on the hearing-impaired individual but on the spouse as well. Emphasis is placed on teaching good communication skills—everything from learning not to start a conversation from another room, to getting rid of other sources of noise by turning off the dishwasher or TV.

In cases of people with more profound hearing loss audiologists spend their time working with both teaching the person to utilize what little hearing he or she has and working with other systems to help with speech and how to get along without hearing. Audiologists work with lip reading skills, sign language, and some simple devices such as a light in place of doorbell, telephone, or alarm clock tones. The audiologist would have knowledge of these devices and be able to make them available to clients.

Teaching

The old saying that 'those who can, do, those who can't, teach' doesn't apply here. In order for someone to become an instructor/professor in a university communication disorders program, he or she must have first become a certified speech-language pathologist or audiologist and fulfilled all the requisite hours for practicing in the field. Those who return to the classroom after a stint in practice bring with them a wealth of hands-on experience in addition to their theoretical knowledge.

A Ph.D. is the usual requirement for entry into university teaching in a communications disorders program, as well as demonstrating an interest in guiding and supervising student therapists.

There is a nationwide shortage of certified speech-language pathologists and audiologists, so there is an increased demand for more teachers who can, in turn, turn out more qualified personnel.

Research

There are those who, rather than practice or teach, are more interested in a career in research. They are fascinated by the different problems human communication presents and work to find solutions to prevent, identify, assess, or rehabilitate speech, language, or hearing disorders.

Areas of interest for researchers include:

- Investigating the physical, biological, and physiological factors underlying normal communication

- Exploring the impact of social, psychological, and psychophysiological factors on communication disorders

- Cooperating with other professionals such as engineers, physicians, and educators to develop a comprehensive approach to working with people with communication disorders

Researchers are most often affiliated with universities and divide their time between classroom teaching and working on various research questions. The usual requirement for a research scientist is a minimum of a Ph.D. degree.

Some research scientists work in industrial settings, for pharmaceutical companies, or for manufacturers of hearing aids or computers.

JOB SETTINGS

Medical Clinics and Hospitals

Therapists working in a medical clinic or hospital setting come in contact with a wide variety of people with a wide variety of disorders. They are able to establish close relationships with their clients because they work with them over a period of time. The relationship usually begins from the point before they've had the cause of the disorder diagnosed, through the diagnosis, treatment, and therapy.

Therapists in this setting also get to work closely with other professionals—physicians, nurses, in some cases neurology professionals, psychologists, physical therapists—to collaborate on effective treatment plans.

Nursing Homes/Rehab Centers

In nursing homes and rehabilitation centers therapists work with elderly patients or patients who have recovered enough from their stroke or injury to be released from the hospital, but are not yet independent enough to return home. Work duties consist mainly of diagnosing and carrying out treatment plans.

Public and Private Schools

In public and private schools the speech-language pathologist works with children, most commonly treating them in a group situation. Children with similar problems would be excused from their regular classrooms for an hour, two or three times a week, to work on particular speech disorders.

Some speech-language pathologists are based at one school; others travel to several different schools within the district. In a school setting, screening for hearing impairment is usually done by the school nurse; the audiologist works more with diagnosis and therapy.

State Schools for the Deaf and Similar Institutions

In state schools for the deaf and similar institutions, therapists work with a more narrow range of problems. Students would all be deaf or perhaps deaf and blind. Students and therapists would meet on a more regular basis than in public or private school settings and the work would focus mainly on improving speech skills.

Working with completely deaf children or deaf and blind children is by far the most challenging—and for some the most rewarding—area of the communication disorders field.

Private Practice

Speech-language pathologists and audiologists can carve out an excellent career for themselves in private practice. Their services are covered by insurance and they can visit clients in their homes or set up their own offices and take referrals from hospitals, ear, nose, and throat (ENT) specialists, and other professionals in the medical community.

Because the schools don't have enough staff to see all the students they have identified with communication disorders, private practitioners also receive referrals through the school board. And during the summer months when schools are closed, parents might take their child to a private practice speech-language pathologist to carry on the therapy started during the regular school year.

Home Health Care Agencies

Home health care agencies operate on both local and national levels. A therapist or audiologist signed up with a local agency will be given assignments as requests come in. National agencies are used by hospitals and other concerns all over the country and provide an opportunity for a practitioner to travel to different cities on short- or long-term assignments.

Colleges and Universities

Some experienced speech-language pathologists and audiologists choose to work in an academic setting, teaching students preparing for careers in communication disorders or conducting research.

TRAINING AND QUALIFICATIONS

Just as with other communications programs, programs in speech-language pathology and audiology can be housed in a number of different university departments with a number of different names and degrees conferred. Commonly, programs are called communication disorders, communicative disorders, communication science, speech communications, speech pathology, and speech-language and hearing pathology. The program name preferred by ASHA is Communication Sciences and Disorders. Degrees conferred could be a Master of Science, Master of Arts, or Master of Education.

The American Speech-Language-Hearing Association certifies speech-language pathologists and audiologists who have met certain criteria. To become certified and awarded a Certificate of Clinical Competence in Speech-Language Pathology (CCC-SLP) or a Certificate of Clinical Competence in Audiology (CCC-A), or certificates in both areas, candidates must:

- Earn a master's degree covering the requisite number of credit hours from an institution whose program is accredited by the Educational Standard Board of the American Speech-Language-Hearing Association

- Complete the requisite number of hours in a supervised clinical observation and a supervised clinical practicum. The practicum cannot be undertaken until sufficient coursework for such an experience has been completed

• Complete a Clinical Fellowship of at least 36 weeks of full-time professional experience or its part-time equivalent in a variety of settings

The master's degree in speech pathology and audiology entails at least 350 hours of clinical contact with patients or clients with communication disorders.

Following the master's program, the final step in completing certification is the successful participation in and completion of a clinical fellowship year. Often the first nine months of your job working full time can be considered as your clinical fellowship year. During that time you would have a certified speech-language pathologist supervising your work. If you were working only half time, it would take you longer to complete the clinical fellowship year.

The clinical fellowship gives you a chance to integrate all you have learned through coursework and the clinical practicum. Bachelor's degree programs are available in communication disorders and many have coursework designed to mesh with a master's program. However, a B.A. in speech-language pathology or communication disorders is not required to enter a master's program in speech-language pathology.

Because of the shortage of certified communication disorders specialists, some bachelor's-level pathologists do find work. But the only setting in which they can be employed with just a bachelor's degree is within different public school systems in some states. They must, however, sign a contract promising to get their master's within four to seven years.

They are allowed to work toward the master's while they are employed, but that can be problematic. Most people working within the public schools are on duty during the times that graduate courses are offered. Some night courses are available, but in some states the programs are not currently designed to accommodate the schedule of working students.

In addition to the coursework, you need between 350 and 375 contact hours in a practicum experience, some of which must be acquired in several different settings working with different types of disorders and different age groups. If you are in the public schools the logistics become very difficult.

Some employed B.A.-level pathologists take a sabbatical from their job to be able to finish. Most find going straight for the master's degree without working to be the most efficient method.

ASHA publishes a handbook that specifies the exact requirements for professional certification. You can contact ASHA at the address listed at the end of this chapter.

Currently 39 states legally require individuals who engage in private practice or who work in non-public agencies to hold a license in speech-language pathology or audiology. Generally, the requirements are similar to those for ASHA certification.

ASHA maintains a list of all state licensing boards and of all accredited university programs in speech-language pathology and audiology.

JOB OUTLOOK

Projections are that job openings will outstrip the supply of qualified candidates for the next ten years. The American Speech-Language-Hearing Association (ASHA) in 1994 prepared a report announcing that shortages of speech-language pathologists and audiologists continue, especially in school settings.

The American Hospital Association (AHA) reports chronic shortages in key hospital occupations including speech-language pathologists. In 1991 one out of every ten speech-language pathologist positions remained unfilled and the vacancies continue.

This is all very good news for future speech-language pathologists and audiologists. Not only are plum jobs waiting for you upon graduation, money is now available to see you through training. In an attempt to meet the need for more trained professionals, scholarship programs have been set up throughout the country on local and state levels as well as through individual university graduate programs. Some of these programs guarantee employment upon graduation.

To find out more about the various scholarships that are available, check with ASHA, local school boards, or graduate communication disorders programs at universities.

Finding Jobs

Communication disorders majors won't need much help locating a job. Because of the shortage of certified speech-language pathologists and audiologists, graduates will find they have their choice of geographic location and job setting. However, to make sure you don't miss hearing about any of the best slots, there are some avenues you can pursue to keep yourself informed.

The American Speech-Language-Hearing Association maintains a computerized placement service and job openings are regularly announced in the professional journals.

Many university departments also hold career days and job fairs, inviting employers from around the country to meet with students and conduct mini-interviews right on the spot.

If you already have a preference for setting and geographic location, you can call the individual personnel departments and let them know of your interest.

SALARIES

Because of the shortage of certified speech-language pathologists and audiologists mentioned earlier, salaries in this career path are very good and are on the rise. The American Speech-Language-Hearing Association (ASHA) conducts an annual salary survey of its members. The most current figures available at this writing are reported from 1993 earnings, which show a 2.9 percent increase from 1992 for certified speech-language pathologists and a 3.4 percent increase from 1992 for audiologists. The median annual salary for speech-language pathologists in 1992 was $34,000 and in 1993 was $35,000. Audiologists earned a median annual salary of $35,782 in 1992 and $37,000 in 1993.

Here are a few other points to consider about salaries in this field:

- Salaries could jump from $28,000 or $30,000 up to $40,000 to $45,000 after the clinical fellowship year depending upon where you work.

- After a few years salaries could go to $60,000 or higher.

- Speech-language pathologists or audiologists working in a school system are usually paid on the same scale as teachers.

- According to a survey conducted by the American Hospital Association, more than 70 percent of the hospitals polled reported that the lack of available candidates is the greatest deterrent to successful recruitment. Hospital human resources executives said that raising salaries is their most common recruitment and retention technique.

- Salaries for college and university instructors and professors generally run much lower than those working in the field. It is not unusual for a professor to see a new student graduate and land a job paying more than he or she is earning.

RELATED FIELDS

Workers in other rehabilitation occupations include occupational therapists, physical therapists, recreational therapists, and rehabilitation counselors.

INTERVIEW

Fay Dudley
Speech-Language Pathologist

Fay Dudley is a speech-language pathologist and is also the supervisor of the speech-language pathology department at a small community hospital. She has been in the field for close to 15 years.

What the Job's Really Like

"I work with adult neurological patients and voice patients, primarily. In addition I do administrative work.

"The neurological patients have had damage, usually as a result of a stroke or hemorrhage or a head trauma of some sort. The voice patients range from people who have been diagnosed with cancer and have had their larynx removed, or they have vocal cord nodules or polyps, or just general vocal cord abuse. These patients talk a lot or talk quickly and empathetically, or are smokers.

"I work Monday through Friday, 8:00 to 4:30. I spend between 30 minutes to an hour with each patient, depending on what the patient can tolerate and what he or she requires. I probably see five or six patients a day. Then I do the administrative work the rest of the time. I have three other speech-language pathologists whom I supervise and, occasionally, we hire per diem therapists, therapists who come in on an as-needed basis, depending on how busy the caseload is.

"I treat outpatients the majority of the time, but if we're short on staff, I'll treat inpatients, too.

"When a patient has actually followed through with my suggestions and I can see progress or hear the changes, that's the most rewarding part of my job.

"And we're lucky enough here to get state-of-the-art equipment related to voice. One of the newest things in the field is doing something called videostroboscopy. You can observe how an individual's vocal cords function and actually see the movement of the cords. And you're also videotaping it at the same time, so you have a record for documentation and review purposes.

"With all the new equipment you can increase your knowledge base and learn. Because, otherwise, if you've been in the field for an extensive period of time, burnout can set in.

"The work, at times, can get monotonous. Once you know the job well, some things are so rote, you don't even have to think about them. When you get an exciting case or something that's different or you're unfamiliar with it, that's great. But most of the cases you get day in and day out are the same. And you get bored.

"As a result, some people leave the field, or sometimes they just accept that it's part and parcel of the job. And there are always times when it's worse, and times when it's better. To keep it interesting you just have to try to expand your horizons or get into new areas of the field. You can work in a different setting or with a different population. One of the things we do that's different is occasionally we work with foreign accent reduction. But we don't get much call for it because it's considered cosmetic and it's not covered by insurance. And therapy is expensive."

How Fay Dudley Got Started

"I had been in business before, in a position where I made decisions and handed decisions down, but there wasn't too much people contact. The main component that led me to this profession was having a lot of people contact and being able to help people.

"I also had a niece who was deaf from meningitis at nine months of age and so that got me thinking about deaf education or speech pathology. I started reading on the subject and thought everything was interesting and that maybe I could get into that.

"I went to the University of Connecticut for a semester on a nondegree status to take some basic courses and to see if I liked it. I already had a bachelor's degree in French and political science, so I went for a master's in speech-language pathology in 1979 and I finished in 1981.

"I ended up working for a corporation that had several contracts with nursing homes. I worked in Pennsylvania with them for two years, then I opened up the Florida division for them. In 1985 I joined the staff of a community hospital. In 1993 I was promoted to supervisor."

Expert Advice

"You need to want to work with people, but you have to recognize that there is emotional stress involved. You have patients who make progress and patients who don't. Some patients you can get involved with and if they don't progress, it's so frustrating for them. And you can definitely sympathize with them because you see that frustration. And that can be emotionally draining on you.

"Overall, I think it's a good field and I've enjoyed it. Again, I think that's because I haven't been stagnant, I've been able to do various things in it. It helps to be independent and organized.

And if you have that quest for knowledge it will help you stay in the field.

"And to know if it's really the field for you, it helps to do observation. Actually go in and watch a speech therapist do therapy. And see a variety of cases, children and adults.

"To find someone you can observe, you can call the national organization or call a local hospital, or even look in the Yellow Pages under speech-language pathology. Check out the different settings. More often than not, whoever's in charge is very willing and open for someone to come in and observe."

● ● ●

FOR MORE INFORMATION

ASHA is the main professional association for speech-language pathologists and audiologists. It has more than 67,000 members and certificate holders and recognizes 52 state speech and hearing association affiliates.

It provides certification to qualified speech-language pathologists and audiologists and accreditation to qualifying university programs.

American Speech-Language-Hearing Association (ASHA)
10801 Rockville Pike
Rockville, MD 20852

Council for Better Hearing and Speech Month
1616 H Street, NW
Washington, DC 20006

National Student Speech-Language-Hearing Association
10801 Rockville Pike
Rockville, MD 20852

Telecommunications for the Deaf
8719 Colesville Road #300
Silver Spring, MD 20910

CHAPTER 11 Funeral Directors

EDUCATION

H.S. Required
Some College Required
Other

$$$ SALARY/EARNINGS

$25,000 to $80,000

OVERVIEW

Since the earliest of times, most peoples have held funeral ceremonies. The dead have ritually been interred in pyramids, cremated on burning pyres, and sunk beneath the oceans' waves. Even today, funeral practices and rites vary greatly among various cultures and religions.

Among the many diverse groups in the United States, funeral practices generally share some common elements: removal of the remains of the deceased to a mortuary, preparation of the remains, performance of a ceremony that honors the deceased and addresses the spiritual needs of the living as well as the dead, and the burial or destruction of the remains. To unburden themselves of arranging and directing these tasks, grieving families turn to funeral directors.

Funeral directors are also called morticians or undertakers. Although this career does not appeal to everyone, the men and women who work as funeral directors take great pride in the fact that they provide efficient and appropriate services that give comfort to their customers.

Funeral directors interview the family to learn what they desire with regard to the nature of the funeral, the clergy members or other persons who will officiate, and the final disposition of the remains; sometimes the deceased leave detailed instructions for their own funerals. Directors establish with the family the location, dates, and times of wakes, memorial services, and burials. They also send a hearse to carry the body to the funeral home or mortuary.

Burial in a casket is the most common method of disposing of remains in this country, although entombments also occur. Cremation, which is the burning of a body in a special furnace, is increasingly selected. Even when remains are cremated, the ashes are often placed in an urn and buried. Funeral directors usually stock a selection of caskets and urns for families to purchase.

Directors arrange the details and handle the logistics of funerals. They prepare obituary notices and have them placed in newspapers, arrange for pallbearers and clergy, schedule with the cemetery the opening and closing of a grave, decorate and prepare the sites of all services, and provide for the transportation of the remains, mourners, and flowers between sites. They also direct preparation and shipment of remains for out-of-state burial.

Funeral services may take place in the home, a house of worship, or the funeral home and at the grave site or crematory. Services may be nonreligious, but often they reflect the religion of the family, so funeral directors must be familiar with the funeral and burial customs of many faiths, ethnic groups, and fraternal organizations. For example, members of some religions seldom have the bodies of the deceased embalmed or cremated.

Most funeral directors are also trained, licensed, and practicing embalmers. In large funeral homes, an embalming staff of one or more embalmers, plus several apprentices, may be employed. Embalming is a sanitary, cosmetic, and preservative process through which the body is prepared for interment. If more than 24 hours or so elapses between death and interment, state laws usually require that remains be embalmed. The embalmer washes the body with germicidal soap and replaces the blood with embalming fluid to preserve the body. Embalmers may reshape and reconstruct disfigured or maimed bodies using materials such as clay, cotton, plaster of Paris, and wax. They also may apply cosmetics to provide a natural appearance, and then dress the body and place it in a casket. Embalmers may maintain records, such as itemized lists of clothing or valuables delivered with the body and the name of the person embalmed.

Funeral directors also handle the paperwork involved with the person's death. They may help family members apply for veterans' burial benefits, notify the Social Security Administration of the death, apply on behalf of survivors for the transfer of any pensions or annuities, and submit papers to state authorities so that a formal certificate of death may be issued and copies distributed to heirs.

Funeral directors are also responsible for the success and the profitability of their businesses. Directors keep records on expenses, purchases, and services rendered; prepare and send invoices for services; prepare and submit reports for unemployment insurance; prepare federal, state, and local tax forms; and prepare itemized bills for customers. Directors also strive to foster a cooperative spirit and friendly attitude among employees and a compassionate demeanor toward the families.

Most funeral homes have a chapel, one or more viewing rooms, a casket-selection room, and a preparation room. Equipment may include a hearse, a flower car, limousines, and sometimes an ambulance.

Funeral directors often work long, irregular hours. Shift work is sometimes necessary because funeral home hours include evenings and weekends. In smaller funeral homes, working hours vary, but in larger homes employees generally work eight hours a day, five or six days a week.

Funeral directors occasionally come into contact with the remains of persons who had contagious diseases, but the possibility of infection is remote if strict health regulations are followed.

To show proper respect and consideration for the families and the dead, funeral directors must dress appropriately. The profession usually requires short, neat haircuts and trim beards, if any, for men. Suits, ties, and dresses are customary for a conservative look.

TRAINING

Funeral directors must be licensed in all but one state, Colorado. Licensing laws vary from state to state, but most require applicants to be 21 years old, have a high school diploma, complete some college training in mortuary science, and serve an apprenticeship. After passing a state board licensing examination, new funeral directors may join the staff of a funeral home.

Embalmers are required to be licensed in all states, and some states issue a single license for both funeral directors and embalmers. In states that have separate licensing and apprenticeship requirements for the two positions, most people in the field obtain both licenses. Persons interested in a career as a funeral director should contact their state board for specific state requirements.

College programs in mortuary science usually last from one to four years, depending on the school. There were 40 mortuary science programs accredited by the American Board of Funeral Service Education in 1994. One-year mortuary science programs offered by some vocational schools emphasized basic subjects such as anatomy, physiology, embalming techniques, and restorative art. Two-year programs were offered by a small number of community and junior colleges, and a few colleges and universities offered both two- and four-year programs.

Longer mortuary science programs included courses in business management, accounting, and use of computers in funeral home management and client services. They also included courses in the social sciences and legal, ethical, and regulatory subjects, such as psychology, grief counseling, oral and written communication, funeral service law, business law, and ethics.

The National Foundation of Funeral Service offers a continuing education program designed for active practitioners in the field. It is a three-week program in communications, counseling, and management. Some states have continuing education requirements that funeral directors must meet before a license can be renewed.

Apprenticeships must be completed under an experienced and licensed funeral director or embalmer. Depending on state regulations, apprenticeships last from one to two years and may be served before, during, or after mortuary school. They provide practical experience in all facets of the funeral service from embalming to transporting remains.

State board licensing examinations vary, but they usually consist of written and oral parts and include a demonstration of practical skills. Persons who want to work in another state may have to pass the examination for that state, although many states will grant licenses to funeral directors from another state without further examination.

High school students can start preparing for a career as a funeral director by taking courses in biology and chemistry and participating in public speaking or debating clubs. Part-time or summer jobs in funeral homes consist mostly of maintenance and clean-up tasks, such as washing and polishing limousines and hearses, but these tasks can help students become familiar with the operation of funeral homes.

Important personal traits for funeral directors are composure, tact, and the ability to communicate easily with the public. They also should have the desire and ability to comfort people in their time of sorrow.

Advancement opportunities are best in large funeral homes at which directors and embalmers may earn promotions to higher-paying positions such as branch manager or general manager. Some directors eventually acquire enough money and experience to establish their own funeral businesses.

JOB OUTLOOK

Funeral directors held about 26,000 jobs in 1994. About one in eight were self-employed. Nearly all worked in the funeral service and crematory industry, but a few worked for the federal government.

Employment of funeral directors and embalmers is expected to increase about as fast as the average for all occupations through the year 2005. Employment opportunities are expected to be excellent, because the number of graduates in mortuary science is likely to continue to be less than the number of job openings in the field.

Demand for funeral services will rise as the population grows, and with it the number of deaths. The population is projected to become older because the number of persons age 55 and over is expected to increase significantly faster than the population as a whole. Deaths will also increase among younger members of the population due to AIDS.

Cremations have been increasing over the years. This trend may lessen the demand for embalming somewhat, because in some states, embalming is not required before cremation. As a consequence, fewer services would be needed from funeral directors.

SALARIES

Salaries of funeral directors depend on the size of the establishment and the number of services performed. A survey conducted by the National Funeral Directors Association found that the average salary, including bonuses, for funeral directors who were owner/managers was $62,506 in 1994; mid-level managers averaged $44,062. Embalmers had average salaries of $27,421, and apprentices averaged $17,489.

RELATED FIELDS

The job of a funeral director requires tact, discretion, and compassion when dealing with grieving people. Others who need these qualities include members of the clergy, social workers, psychologists, psychiatrists, and other health care professionals.

●   ●   ●

INTERVIEW
R. Todd Noecker
Funeral Director and Embalmer

R. Todd Noecker is a past president of the Wyoming Funeral Directors Association. He is a certified Wyoming coroner and a licensed funeral director and embalmer in both Wyoming and Arizona. He has an A.A. from the University of Wyoming in Laramie, with courses in business administration and a degree in mortuary science from the

Dallas Institute of Mortuary Science in Texas. He is one of three funer-al directors at Mt. View Memorial Gardens in Mesa, Arizona. He has been in this profession since 1982.

What the Job's Really Like

"Funeral directing is a career that carries many job titles—a maintenance person of sorts, most funeral directors are responsible for the lawn mowing, car washing, vacuuming, and overall appearance of the funeral home. We're grief counselors for families following a death, and explaining to them the aspects and details of a funeral service at a time when comprehending all of this is very hard.

"We're legal secretaries, in that we compile all the information needed for a death certificate. We file these with the county and state agencies as well as notifying Social Security, Veterans Administration, workers' compensation, or Railroad Retirement. We also notify insurance companies of a death if a family chooses.

"We're accountants, too, in that we compile all charges for the family and complete a statement of funeral goods and services.

"We're writers in that we compose the obituaries and send them to the newspaper the family chooses.

"We also act as an agent, contacting outside sources for the family such as clergy, musicians, police escorts, and veterans associations for deceased veterans. We also handle all arrangements with the cemetery the family chooses.

"We're decorators in that we arrange all the flowers (possibly three or more times) for the funeral service. There are many other smaller details too numerous to mention. But above all else we are very good listeners.

"Basically, I meet with families following a death, gather information regarding the deceased and the type of funeral services the family is requesting.

"Most funeral directors are embalmers as well. Embalming is the chemical sanitation of a human body. It is somewhat like a postmortem surgical procedure. It allows families time for a public visitation by preserving the body for the funeral services. Embalmers and funeral directors alike also dress the body in clothing usually brought in by the family as well as take care of the cosmetizing and hairdressing of the deceased.

"The hours are the downside. I'm on call 24 hours a day, seven days a week. It can be very nerve-racking. It takes a lot of control and self-discipline to awaken in the middle of the night, dress and go to a family's home where a death has occurred and speak with them, then take the deceased back to the mortuary for preparation.

"I believe it is a very important profession, vital to the communities we serve, as well as vital to the families' well-being with whom we work."

How R. Todd Noecker Got Started

"I am a fourth-generation funeral director, originally from Gillette, Wyoming. I was brought up in the death care industry—born into the profession like many other funeral directors.

My father and grandfather were both coroners as well as funeral directors. The state of Wyoming says that you should have at least two years of liberal arts plus be a graduate of an accredited college of mortuary science. Following this you must successfully pass the National Board of Funeral Service Exam, as well as your state licensing exams—both the funeral service and embalmers portions.

"I have attended well over 200 hours of continuing education courses pertaining to grief counseling, homicide investigation, modes of death, dealing with suicide, infant death, and many other types of death, which are difficult cases and of course devastating to families.

"I don't own my own business now, but I did once before. Where I work there are three other funeral directors besides myself."

Expert Advice

"Make sure that you are sincere about the profession you are about to embark on. It takes a very special, professional, caring, and dedicated person to be a funeral director.

"You must have very good people skills in order to deal with the public and good business skills to deal with the inventory of caskets, printed materials, and daily operations. It is a position that requires a well-rounded individual who can attend to all the various details.

"This profession demands much of your time and your energy, as well as your emotions. Explore, explore, explore. If in the end you find yourself drawn to the profession, it is one of great pride."

●　　●　　●

FOR MORE INFORMATION

Information on a career as a funeral director is available from:

The National Funeral Directors Association
11121 West Oklahoma Avenue
Milwaukee, WI 53227

National Selected Morticians
1616 Central Street
Evanston, IL 60201

For a list of accredited programs in mortuary science and scholarship information contact:

The American Board of Funeral Service Education
14 Crestwood Road
Cumberland, ME 04021

For information on continuing funeral service education contact:

The National Foundation of Funeral Service
2250 East Devon Avenue, Suite 250
Des Plaines, IL 60018

About the Author

Blythe Camenson's main concern as a full-time writer of career books is helping job seekers make educated choices. She firmly believes that with enough information, readers can find long-term, satisfying careers. To that end, she researches traditional as well as unusual occupations, talking to a variety of professionals about what their jobs are really like. In all of her books she includes firsthand accounts from people who can reveal what to expect in each occupation, the upsides as well as the down.

Camenson's interests range from history and photography to writing novels. She is also director of Fiction Writer's Connection, a membership organization providing support to new and published writers.

Camenson was educated in Boston, earning her B.A. in English and psychology from the University of Massachusetts and her M.Ed. in counseling from Northeastern University.

In addition to *On the Job: Real People Working in the Helping Professions*, other books she has written for NTC/Contemporary Publishing Company are:

Career Portraits: Travel

Career Portraits: Writing

Career Portraits: Nursing

Career Portraits: Firefighting

Careers for History Buffs

Careers for Plant Lovers

Careers for Health Nuts

Careers for Mystery Buffs

Careers for Self-Starters

Great Jobs for Art Majors

Great Jobs for Communications Majors

Great Jobs for Liberal Arts Majors

On the Job: Real People Working in Service Businesses

On the Job: Real People Working in Health Care

On the Job: Real People Working in Sales and Marketing

On the Job: Real People Working in Education

On the Job: Real People Working in Law Careers

On the Job: Real People Working in Engineering

Opportunities in Museum Careers

Opportunities in Teaching English to Speakers of Other Languages

Opportunities in Zoo Careers